MW01152735

VAGUS NERVE: Shield Against C-Spine, Balance Loss, Dizziness, and Clouded Mind

Discover the Healing Secrets of the Vagus Nerve, Meditation, and Polyvagal Theory to Treat Neck Pain

Written by:

Emma Gentile

application of the contents of this book, directly or indirectly, in breach of a contract, through wrong, negligence, personal injury, criminal intent, or under any other circumstance.

You agree to accept all risks arising from the use of the information presented in this book.

You agree that, by continuing to read this book, when appropriate and/or necessary, you will consult a professional (including, but not limited to, your doctor, lawyer, financial advisor, or other such professional) before using the remedies, techniques or the information suggested in this book.

Table of Contents

Introduction

Welcome to! I am very happy that you are reading these words. This book was born with the dual intention of letting you know about the tools you have at your disposal every day to fight stress, anxiety, and emotional situations that make you breathless, how to make the most of them, and face everyday life with a different spirit. By doing research and listening to people, I realized more concretely that the Vagus Nerve performs numerous functions that are also useful for relieving chronic pain that affects those who suffer from neck pain. This is why I wanted to deepen both topics, making you understand how many elements typical of one actually influence the other more or less directly. Stress, anxiety, muscle stiffness, migraine, and dizziness affect not only the Vagus Nerve but also the cervical spine; vice versa, if you have been suffering from neck pain for decades, can't find a remedy and change pillows or spend a fortune on massages, just be aware that in the Vagus Nerve you have found a resource and a source of energy that you can activate at any time with a little practice: in the office, while playing in the park with your children or when you are having dinner with a friend with wet hair and *here it is!* An excruciating head pain that responds by making you vomit or giving you the feeling of being in a boat at the slightest movement! For this (and many other reasons) I have collected numerous bibliographic resources that allow you to learn what the Vagus Nerve is, where it is and what functions it performs, which branches of the nervous system are active and when, more than 25 ways to activate it and which ones can be the situations to avoid. You can appreciate the correlation with the cervical spine by learning 11 techniques to manage chronic pain, relaxation, and meditation techniques, the vertebrae and muscle groups involved and what functions they perform, examples of specific exercises + BONUS online resources. As you can already see from the index, there are many topics and I have tried to prepare them for you in a simple and effective way. I hope you will appreciate them!

Enjoy your reading!

Part 1

Why the C-Spine Pain Is Different From a Normal Pain

As mentioned in the introduction, to understand the functions and importance of the Vagus Nerve and its correlations with a cervical disorder, I find it interesting to understand why the latter bursts during a walk, while we are having dinner with friends and suddenly you have excruciating pangs that spread from one side of the head to the other and almost make you lose your balance, your head seems to become a boulder (we will understand why), dizziness, you see everything blurred and your ears seem as muffled as if you just did a freediving competition ... *do I have to continue?! No, I think these are sensations you know too well!* This is because the cervical tract is very complex, and it would be useful to know a little more about it. Its complexity is given by the fact that it has muscle bands, cranial nerves (including the X cranial nerve, or the Vagus Nerve), various vertebrae, and countless structures and nerve endings that are fundamental to carry out even the most trivial actions and whose gears are perfect. However, a bit like the New York road network that sees thousands of people and cabs jammed into its lanes at rush hour; it is normal for some clogging to occur when the system is subjected to intense stresses. The same metaphor represents our habits, the physical and emotional stresses that daily, due to or thanks to our lifestyle, are reflected on our whole body and also on the cervical tract. Physically demanding workloads, difficult emotions to manage, anxiety, etc. cause a state of general stress that is also reflected on the muscles in difficulty because they are not trained and which, with different timing for each of us, also lead to cervical problems since they often cannot bear the load that we impose on them (Chiapponi, 2020). So, if you understand something more about the articulated structure of the cervical tract, about the important functions that the Vagus Nerve performs, which will be explored in the next sections *(don't worry, you don't need a degree in medicine!)*, the role played by the activities you do and the role of the activities that you do not do every day out of laziness, because you do not know them or because you think you are not able, you will acquire a great awareness that combined with the experience of a professional, whose work is fundamental, will make you understand potential that you have at your fingertips and that every day is at your disposal to help you implement empowering habits and achieve long-term benefits that will improve the quality of your life. In the next section, you will learn about a widespread false myth about the cervical spine and you will understand some tricks that will allow you to ease the tension on this part of your body.

The False Myth About the C-Spine

It Is All About Posture

Let's start by framing a well-known problem and then understand how the Vagus Nerve can help us in this, where it is located, and what functions it has. A statement you often hear is that neck pain depends a lot on incorrect posture, but why do we consider posture so important? What is actually meant by this term? In this regard, a very authoritative source in this field is Paul Ingraham, who on his site painscience.com has collected years of experience and knowledge in this field and beyond. According to his ten-year observations, he believes that many people, especially those with a strong awareness and interest in the person's well-being at 360 degrees, must somehow "correct" their posture since incorrect positions have become consolidated habits over the years, they have led them to have very common problems including neck pain, headache, and back pain. Surely the way we sit, stand and the pace with which we walk are rooted not only in the years but also in our personality (Ingraham, 2021). As explained in the article, there is in fact what is called "poor posture" or a set of postural habits at the basis of physical stress that becomes chronic as the years pass and that could actually be avoided, but not only. First of all, what is meant by posture? Contrary to what is commonly thought, it is not a specific position, but a dynamic pattern of reflexes, habits, and responses that our body adopts in reference to the environment that surrounds it and that "challenges" the body's ability to maintain a standing and functioning position, i.e., factors such as:

- Gravity.
- Particular and unavoidable positions that you assume while you work (e.g. a nurse cannot fail to lift patients to take care of them), or self-imposed positions using chairs or other low-quality ergonomic tools.
- Particular anatomy.
- Athletic challenges.

So it is clear that the concept is much more complex than you have always thought: it is the way you live that shapes your body through certain movements. These, very often, are the mirror of your social interactions and your emotional needs that derive from them, when you feel comfortable or uncomfortable depending on the situation, movements that you will tend to repeat or rather avoid. A posture can indicate openness or closure, happiness or sadness, courage or fear depending on the contexts you live. Changing posture, therefore, does not only involve the musculoskeletal part of your body but is a profound process. The patterns and behaviors that cause illness, therefore, require more understanding and effort to change. So, what is the importance of posture? In a 2019 study, several hundred professionals were asked how important it was for them to assume a correct sitting and standing posture: as many as 65% considered this to be "very" important and 28% "quite" important; however several opinions remained discordant since they were not based on scientific evidence. So, how should we consider the posture topic? You can consider it as one of the many factors that contribute to making you feel pain; sometimes, however, it is not about that. This is true if you consider the fact that there are people who pay particular attention to posture and suffer from a lot of pain and others who do not take particular care of it and do not suffer from any disturbance. Another widespread belief: keeping the shoulders and upper part of the back curved causes pain. It's not a cure-all, but to disprove this cause-and-effect relationship, ten different experiments and a very large study dating back to 1994 on kyphosis reported that not even 10% of the participants suffered from particularly severe pain.

Postural Stress vs. Incorrect Posture

A topic that is rarely talked about is the difference between bad posture and postural stress; the latter represents a kind of "challenge" with respect to the posture you usually hold, partly out of habit and partly out of boredom and this too varies according to the moment you are experiencing. Here are some examples (Ingraham, 2021):

- Trying to sleep does not require straining the neck in strange positions in completely uncomfortable contexts such as the back seat of a car or plane.
- A nurse has to bend over the patients and perform particular positions to lift them or for other tasks.

Sometimes postural stress and poor posture overlap. An example is carrying a very heavy package on one shoulder: sometimes it is necessary but the decision to load the package on your shoulder is yours. So your role in this action is active. So, why do some people suffer and others don't? Although the human body is able to withstand a certain degree of asymmetry; sometimes in cases of lighter pain, we speak more of vulnerability to the pain itself rather than posture itself. A vulnerability, subjective pain sensitivity that inevitably increases with age and makes you the subject of inflammation.

A "Good" Posture

You can consider it as a dynamic approach that promotes movement over a sedentary lifestyle. There's no need to overdo it, but a little more movement is a great start. We conclude this section by stating that in some cases the posture is linked to some problems that cause painful situations; however, it is not as closely related as many people believe (Ingraham, 2021).

A Control Unit of Impulses

As you will remember, we started this explanation by underlining the complex structure of the cervical tract and now we are going to better understand the interactions that exist between it and the Vagus Nerve, or rather... the Vagus Nerves. Well yes, there are two of them, one right and one left. They perform innumerable functions and cause, when too stressed, fatigue, dizziness, inability to concentrate, widespread malaise; do you recognize yourself? Well! Then let's proceed in order.

Vagus Nerve: Where It Is Located

First of all, as explained in the article by Leanage (2020), the Vagus Nerve is the 10th cranial nerve (CN X), originates in the marrow of the brainstem and exits the skull through the jugular foramen together with the Glossopharyngeal Nerve (CN IX) and Accessory nerve (CN XI). Inside the skull, there is also an auditory innervation (Arnold's Nerve) from the superior ganglion of the Vagus Nerve that connects with the auditory canal and external ear. As shown in Figure 1, at the neck the Vagus Nerve crosses the carotid sheath. At the base of the neck, the two Vagus nerves divide and follow different paths: the right Vagus Nerve branches in front of the subclavian artery and behind the sternoclavicular joint, thus entering the chest. The left Vagus Nerve, on the other hand, flows in the lower part, left side of the common carotid, and posterior to the sternoclavicular joint to also enter the chest.

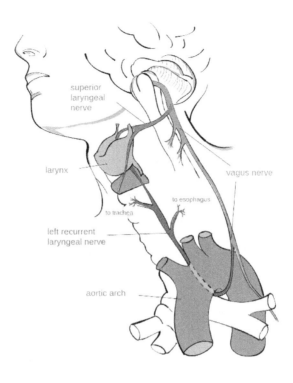

Figure 1: Simplified Overview of the Major Branches of the Vagus Nerve [1]

Three main branches originate from this area:

- **Pharyngeal:** Provides motor innervation to most of the muscles of the pharynx and soft palate.

- **Superior laryngeal nerve:** This is divided into external and internal. The external one innervates the cricothyroid muscles of the larynx; the internal branching innervates the hypopharynx and the upper part of the larynx.

---

[1] Source Figure 1: https://teachmeanatomy.info/head/cranial-nerves/vagus-nerve-cn-x/ This photo by Unknown Author is licensed under CC BY-SA. Created February 5, 2014.

17

- **Recurrent laryngeal nerve (right side only):** From the right side of the subclavian artery, it ascends towards the larynx, innervating most of the muscles present.

In the thorax, the right vagal nerve forms the posterior vagal trunk while the left branch forms the anterior vagal trunk. Some branches here form the esophageal plexus which innervates the smooth muscles of the esophagus. In the abdomen, the vagal trunk ends by dividing into branches that affect not only the esophagus but also the stomach and large intestine. As you will see below, the Vagus Nerve performs a very important function in the intestine.

Vagus Nerve: Its Functions

It constitutes the greater part of the Parasympathetic Nervous System (SNP) which is activated when we are in conditions of relaxation. In those moments, the main functions that the Vagus Nerve performs are (Chiapponi, 2021):

- Promotes muscle recovery and relaxation function.
- Reduces heart rate and controls mood (Breit et al., 2018).
- Promotes digestion by increasing gastric acid and intestinal peristalsis.
- Performs an anti-inflammatory function thanks to the production of acetylcholine (one of the most important neurotransmitters, responsible for central and peripheral nerve transmission).

A function that deserves to be deepened concerns digestion and the role that the Vagus Nerve plays as an informer of the brain regarding what happens in the viscera (Chiapponi, 2021). It follows that if the stomach and/or intestines are constantly inflamed, the Vagus Nerve will also be affected. As explained in Breit et al. (2018), there is two-way communication between the brain and the gastrointestinal tract which constitutes a real axis. Thanks to hormones and enzymes, these act in synergy with the Vagus Nerve to control appetite and food intake. Have you ever heard that the intestine is the second brain? This is exactly the case, as the enteric nervous system (ENS), which is part of the autonomic nervous system, controls the digestive system and is characterized by 100–150 million neurons, the area with the most neurons ever after the brain. The ENS serves as an intestinal barrier that regulates most enteric processes such as the immune response, nutrient detection, intestinal motility (the ability to advance food in the digestive tract), microvascular circulation, and epithelial secretion of fluids. So there is a continuous exchange of information but not only, as the enteric nervous system is at the same time equally independent of the Vagus Nerve as circuits, sensory and motor neurons regulate the activity and motility of various muscles and part of the immune system. Given these functions, you can appreciate how a machine as complex as the human body can benefit from the choices you make every day. In light of what has been said so far, considering the exchange of information that takes place between the intestine and the brain, food choices also contribute to limiting the inflammatory state of your body and, as we will see later, help you find relief for the cervical problem. Although every situation is different, it is worth trying to have some more foresight; so much so that, again the study by Breit et al. (2018), concludes by stating that the correlation between nutrition and the Vagus Nerve is well known and proven. Consider that vagal tone influences weight gain, obesity, and inflammatory stress diseases. Meditation and stimulation of the Vagus Nerve are very useful in this case... but we will have the opportunity to talk about this later! I have a few surprises, just for you!

A Breath of Air and You Immediately Have to Wear a Scarf and Cap?

Discover the Joint Between the Brain and the Cervical Spine

Have you ever been outdoors chatting with friends or taking a walk, and just because of some wind you immediately started feeling pangs? In this section you will learn more about the vertebrae in the cervical spine and why your head sometimes appears to be a boulder. A very important and delicate area of your body is the vertebral skull joint where the transition from the brain to the spine takes place. As indicated in Figure 2, we find a sequence of vertebrae that, from the occipital bone (C0), continues with the first vertebra of the atlas (C1, atlas) in the form of a ring, the second axis vertebrae (C2, axis) to continue up to the seventh vertebra (C7). The occipital bone, the atlas, and the axis are the vertebrae responsible for most of the rotational movements, extension, and flexion capacity of the spine. There is simply no point in your spine that has a superior range of motion (Traynelis, 2020). Traynelis goes on to explain that the occipital bone is the only bone in the skull that connects it with the cervical tract and covers the back of the head called the occiput.

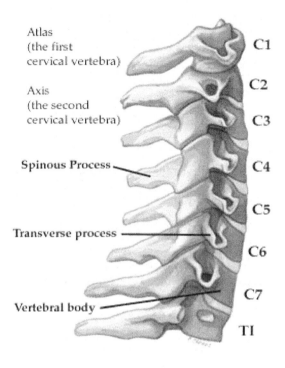

Figure 1: Overview of the vertebrae present in the cervical tract. [2]

Do you remember the myth of Atlas who supported the globe on his shoulders? Yup?! Well, the vertebra of the atlas (C1) seems to get its name from there and it is only thanks to it that you were able to nod with your head to my question; in fact, it acts as a pivot that allows you to move the garment back and forth. This is as trivial as it is impossible when you are

[2] Source Figure 2: This photo by Unknown Author is licensed under CC-BY-SA.
Creation   date   21/01/2016.
https://operativeneurosurgery.com/lib/exe/detail.php?id=cervical_spine&media=cervicalspine.j
pg

hit by the pangs of the cervical. As you can see from Figure 2, after the atlas there is the vertebrae of the axis (C2), which, like the atlas, is distinguished by structure and function from the remaining vertebrae. Between these two there is a synovial joint called the atlantoaxial joint which facilitates rotational movement. The axis is characterized by the presence of a bone called the "tooth" that functions as a peg: that's when you shake your head and say no: that's what allows you to do it! As you can see, it is an extremely important part of your body, vulnerable and complex because it is rich in blood and neurological activity so knowing it allows you to have a greater awareness of what is happening to you (Traynelis, 2020), or at least to have further indications for identify the parties involved and ask more specific questions to your doctor or the professional you decide to contact. Often there can be several problems affecting the C1 and C2 vertebrae (it is in this area that the Vagus Nerve flows), below are some common problems and symptoms that can occur taken from Dickerman (2019). In this interesting article they mention themselves:

- **Arthritis:** An extremely common problem that is divided into different types such as rheumatoid arthritis or rather a form of arthrosis that affects the spine by inflaming it. This condition is due to a high movement of the joint between the atlas and axis; this can eventually lead to nerve root or spinal compression.

- **Fractures:** Usually a fracture of the C1 and C2 vertebrae involves both. The causes are manifold; from swimming in shallow water, a fall, a motorcycle accident, or a bump where you hit your forehead or chin. Nonetheless, we mention whiplash or fractures affecting the spine.

- **Damage to the vertebral arteries:** By supplying the brain, damage of this type can lead to serious neurological consequences.
- **Occipital neuralgia:** Damage to the spinal cord at the level of the C2 vertebra can lead to frequent headaches.
- **Crowned tooth syndrome:** That is when calcium present in the ligaments of the axis is deposited on the tooth of the vertebra itself, causing inflammation and reducing the mobility of the C1-C2 joint.

Dickerman lists several common symptoms and signs and states that they can cause pain of various kinds. You can have light and constant pain with very specific pangs in the cervical spine, it can be a short-lasting pain, rather than a chronic and recurring one. If the nerve root present in the axis becomes inflamed or suffers further damage, other symptoms may occur such as:

- A pain that radiates from the back to the top of the head.
- Pain in the temples and/or in the back of the ears and eyes.
- Numbness or other non-ordinary sensations affecting at least one side of the neck and tongue.
- Sensitivity to light.
- Tiredness and fatigue.
- Nausea.
- Dizziness.

Are they familiar to you? These symptoms usually get worse when you lie down and the pain can also increase at night while you sleep, affecting the quality of your sleep. Dickerman concludes by stating that compression in the C2 area can therefore cause even very severe pain, tingling, numbness and a decrease in sensitivity, weakness in the arms and legs, and sometimes problems with bladder control. In very critical cases it can even be fatal as basic life functions such as breathing can be compromised or stopped.

Vertebrae C2–C5

We continue in the explanation by talking about the characteristics and functions of the three successive vertebral segments: C2–C3, C3–C4, and finally C4–C5. To get to know them, I will share with you some very interesting information explained by Meyler (2019). This section starts from the axis (C2) which we now know very well and ends in the intermediate part of the cervical spine with the C5 vertebra. This segment mostly contributes to the intermediate range of motion when we tilt our heads forward and/or backward. In this set of movements, the C4–C5 segment is typically characterized by a greater movement capacity than the two previous sections. Comparing this section with the C5–C7 vertebrae that we will see later, the latter are more prone to trauma than the C2–C5. However, damage to the C2–C5 segment can cause degeneration, hernias, trauma, and neurological injury. Segment C2–C5 includes the following structures:

- **Vertebrae and joints:** The C2–C5 vertebrae are held together by ligaments and connected by a pair of joints also present in the rest

24

of the vertebral column. In particular, they are of the synovial type and contain inside them the cartilage that helps to "oil" and make the movements between the vertebrae fluid.

- **Intervertebral discs:** Between one vertebra and the other there is a fibrous ring structure inside which there is a sort of gelatinous core that allows to absorb shocks and avoid rubbing between vertebrae during movements, while always allowing movement in all directions.

- **Spinal nerves:** Present within each mobile segment; from the spinal cord, the spinal nerves come out through small bony openings on both sides, right and left, of the vertebral canal. These openings are called intervertebral foramina and are located between two adjacent vertebrae.

Each spinal nerve receives impulses and signals from a specific skin region (called a dermatome, which is a specific area innervated by a single spinal nerve root). At the same time each spinal nerve controls a very specific group of muscles, let's see them together (Meyler 2019):

- **Dermatome involving the C3 vertebra:** In this case, the spinal nerve affects the skin region of the upper part of the neck where there is a part of the musculature that helps the head to lean forward and backward.

- **Dermatome that affects the C4 vertebra:** Usually affects the skin region of the shoulders and consequently the musculature that allows their movement.

- **Dermatome involving the C5 vertebra:** In this case, in addition to the shoulders, the skin regions of the upper arms and forearms are affected. The dermatome of the C5 vertebra also includes some muscles that aid shoulder movements.

Some nerve branches originating in the phrenic nerve and affecting the C3, C4, and C5 vertebrae innervate the diaphragm allowing breathing. Inside the spinal canal of each segment, the spinal cord is protected anteriorly by the vertebral body and posteriorly by the vertebral arch. Here are some common issues affecting this segment:

- **Cervical spondylosis:** Consequent to degeneration due to arthrosis, it leads to wear on the joints that join the vertebrae of the cervical tract.

- **Hernias affecting the discs:** In this case, they can irritate or compress the neighboring nerve root.

- **Fractures:** Due to trauma, falls, motorcycle accidents, or whiplash.

- **Congenital stenosis:** Often occurring at birth.

- **Damage to the phrenic nerve:** It could happen due to more or less direct trauma or due to the presence of spondylosis.

Let's see together the most common symptoms that can affect the problems that I just mentioned. Meyler considers:

- Moderate to very severe pain may be felt in the neck, shoulders, and/or upper arms. The pain can radiate from the upper neck to the back and head causing the typical cervical migraine that can be worsened by moving the neck and/or arms.

- Numbness in one or more parts of the forearm, hands, or fingers.

- Weakness in the shoulders, elbow, and/or wrist makes it more difficult for these joints to move.

- Difficulty in breathing or inability to breathe due to damage to the phrenic nerve.

Vertebrae C5–C6

Here we are at the lower part of the cervical tract which has the task of providing flexibility and support to much of the neck and head (which sometimes looks like a boulder). Thanks to, or because of this load-bearing function that the C5–C6 vertebrae must perform, they are often affected by various kinds of trauma, hernias, a posture that does not help, and radicular pain (Zigler, 2018) which I will explain shortly. Also in this case we find a vertebral structure along the lines of that previously described with a body, a vertebral arch, and a fibrous ring structure between the vertebrae that allows absorbing shocks. It is interesting to briefly describe which muscle bands affect the dermatomes present in this area (Zigler, 2018). In particular, in this case, the dermatome and myomere C6 are mentioned:

- **C6 dermatome:** This skin region affects the upper and lateral area of the thumb and index finger of the hand to go up the forearm and reach above the shoulder, reconnecting to the C6 vertebra.

- **Myomere C6:** That is the muscle band innervated by the single spinal nerve that affects the wrist extensor muscle that allows it to flex backward, the supinator muscle, and the humeral biceps; which allow you to bend the elbow and rotate the forearm.

Also for this cervical tract, it is useful to complete the overview of these vertebrae by mentioning some common problems that may be encountered and some curiosities:

- **Vertebral disc problems:** The presence of hernias, in this case, is very common and it is these two C5-C6 vertebrae that suffer particularly. This is also due to a "*recisive*" effect that discs undergo when you keep your head bowed forward while you are at the PC or while staring at Instagram almost hypnotized; that is, while partly for work needs and partly for leisure, you spend hours in front of the screen without realizing it and in recent years, in fact, the "smartphone syndrome" has become the new cervical, also called "text neck". Nevertheless, other causes of this pain are whiplash or rather the natural aging process that advances with age.

- **Spondylosis:** As mentioned in the previous section, this problem also occurs here. In this tract, however, it manifests itself in a higher percentage and often results in the formation of bone spurs or the restriction of the intervertebral foramen (i.e. the central cavity of the vertebra delimited by the body and vertebral arch).

- **Fractures:** In this case, it is interesting to report some data to better quantify the problem. According to research carried out in this field, as much as 20% of traumatic fractures of the cervical tract occur precisely at the level of the C6 vertebra, while 15% at the C5. In these cases the whiplash blows that force the cervical tract to make a very abrupt movement and which can cause fractures which in turn undermine the stability of the neck and cause injury to the spine, stand out.

- **Congenital stenosis:** In this case, a narrowing and pressure are exerted on the cord and spinal root which has genetic origins.

Before going on to mention the additional symptoms you may encounter, I will focus on a concept introduced earlier, namely root pain. Some information and curiosities (Schenato, 2021): first of all it is a problem that affects the nerve root for an inflammatory or compressive reason. However, with a positive outcome, it is a problem that most frequently affects men between the ages of 50 and 54, and 83 out of 100,000 people are affected. A distinction: we speak of radicular pain when it is caused by some ectopic discharges, which means that an organ or other element is out of place, discharges originating from the dorsal root or ganglion; while we speak of radiculopathy when we refer to a neurological state in which nerve conduction is compromised. While some physiological changes associated with aging can be considered as a cause, on the other, the inflammatory state affecting nearby structures affecting the nervous structures should not be underestimated. These problems can start suddenly or rather increase over time, typically anticipated by pain in the back of the neck and accompanied by decreasing mobility. Also in this case some symptoms, already seen previously, are reported, such as pain on the shoulders, a pain that affects all the components of the arm up to the individual fingers of the hand, rather than stinging that subsequently radiates from the neck inside the arm. Nevertheless, this segment of the cervical tract can also be the origin of a numbness extended to the whole arm to affect the hand and weakness that makes the movement of the shoulders, elbow, and wrist more difficult.

Vertebrae C6–C7

This segment supports the weight that affects both the head and the remaining vertebrae described so far; furthermore, the lower part (C7) is connected to the first vertebra of the thorax (T1). As explained by Levine (2019), the additional problems and symptoms already mentioned in the previous sections are also reflected here, however it is interesting to note some structural differences that distinguish the C6-C7 vertebrae from the previous vertebrae, specifically following differences:

- The key elements of the C6 vertebra in addition to the presence of the arch and the vertebral body, are two transverse processes and one spinous process, and two joint facets (facet). Figure 3 on the next page helps you to better visualize the structure.

The C7 vertebra, on the other hand, is distinguished by some characteristics that make it unique in its own way:

- A more pronounced spinous transversus that can also be perceived at the base of the neck and allows attachment, connection to a greater number of cervical muscle bands than the previous vertebrae.

- The transverse foramen (foramen transversium in Figure 3) in this case does not contain the vertebral artery whose task is to transport blood to the brain, an element present in the remaining vertebrae.

- In exceptional cases, there may be an additional cervical rib whose extremity either ends in the soft tissue, or in the first rib that delimits the upper chest opening.

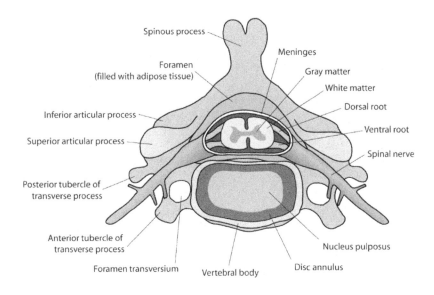

Figure 2: Vertebral structure example. (3)

Before concluding this part, which I hope has helped you to learn more about your body and the origins of possible symptoms that you happen to perceive, let's mention the C7 dermatome and myomere.

---

3 Source Figure 3: https://upload.wikimedia.org/wikipedia/commons/d/d9/Cervical_vertebra_english.png
user: debivort, CC BY-SA 3.0 <http://creativecommons.org/licenses/by-sa/3.0/>, via Wikimedia Commons

- **Dermatome C7:** The spinal nerve in question emerges between the two vertebrae C6 and C7. The dermatome in this case affects the skin region of the shoulders, back, the back of the arms, and the middle finger.

- **Myomere C7:** The muscle band involved in this case is the one that allows you to extend the elbow forward, raise the wrist, stretch the fingers and extend the hand and its triceps connected to it.

Non-Surgical Treatments

In light of what has been said so far, you may be wondering what is possible to do. There are several alternatives, some common to more segments of the cervical tract, while other treatments may be more suitable for some parts rather than others, below is a brief overview starting from the two common practices taken from Dickerman (2019) and Meyler (2019):

- **Physiotherapy:** You have probably already tried it yourself, and it is indicated for strengthening the muscles that surround the vertebrae and improve posture. Physiotherapy carried out for the C1-C2 vertebrae helps to keep the atlanto-occipital part in balance (Dickerman, 2019). In the case of the C2-C5 vertebrae segment, physiotherapy is useful for strengthening the neck muscles, improving posture (remember the dynamic concept of posture seen at the beginning of the book). Physiotherapy activities, carried out under the supervision of a professional, may include stretching or other exercises, massages, or other activities (Meyler, 2019).

- **Traction:** As for the C1–C2 vertebrae, these are exercises of lengthening and/or realigning the spine to relieve the direct pressure of the nerve on the vertebrae, particularly in this segment it can be useful to decrease the compression on the C2 nerve both in adults and children. However, it is an effective treatment only for a limited period of time and therefore provides only temporary relief. It can be done manually or with the aid of appropriate instruments. Also with regard to the segment C2–C5 it can help to relieve and loosen the compression of the spinal nerve.

Now let's see the specific alternatives that Dickerman proposes for the C1–C2 vertebrae:

- **Medicines:** Both prescription and over-the-counter drugs include alternatives that help relax muscles such as non-steroidal anti-inflammatory drugs (NSAIDs).

- **Immobilization:** The use of a collar or neck brace may be recommended in the case of fractures of these two vertebrae, in order to prevent any type of movement and maintain proper alignment of the same.

- **Manipulation:** Performed with chiropractic techniques it can help in some cases to relieve pain; however it is not recommended when the stability of the C1-C2 vertebrae is compromised.

- **Injection of anti-inflammatories:** The injection of anti-inflammatories or other medicines that help reduce pain in the area

33

between the atlanto-occipital joint. They are usually performed using X-ray technology and a radiopaque dye capable of blocking the passage of the same X-rays. Studies have shown that in 80% of cases, more than 50% of patients were able to appreciate a reduction in pain between the C1-C2 vertebrae by 50%.

Let's now see some possibilities for the subsequent cervical tract involving the C2–C5 vertebrae (Meyler, 2019). Basically, you can consider the solutions already mentioned valid, however in this case we can have two different alternatives of minimally invasive injections that are usually not proposed as the first option:

- **Steroid injection:** Or other anesthetizing drugs can be injected into different parts of the vertebra such as the facet joints or the epidural space (space between the dura mater and the yellow ligament, it is a space characterized for example by blood vessels of limited size).
  In particular, thanks to this remedy, people who have suffered whiplash or rather people who suffer from radicular pain seem to benefit.

- **Radiofrequency ablation:** In this case, it involves heating a part of the nerve that transmits pain with a special needle and creating a lesion due to heat that prevents the nerve from transmitting pain signals to the brain. It can be useful for controlling the pain transmitted by the facet joints.

Meyler concludes by pointing out that injections carry a very limited risk of producing a hematoma, bleeding, or nerve damage. The fundamental thing is to get information and always contact a trained specialist.

Vagus Nerve, Headache, and Text Neck

Advantages of Vagus Nerve Stimulation and Areas of Application

By stimulation of the vagus nerve (VNS), we mean the set of techniques that can be used for this purpose, whether they are manual or performed through electrical stimulation. For example, stimulation of the left vagus nerve is a recognized therapy for the treatment of refractory epilepsy (that is, due to problems of the immune system it does not respond to the therapies applied) and for treatment-resistant depressive forms. On the contrary, stimulation of the right vagus nerve is useful in the treatment of heart failure in preclinical studies and the second phase of clinical trials. In the future, it will be possible to have more feedback in this sense (Howland, 2015). The Vagus Nerve is made up of 20% of efferent (motor) fibers that send signals from the brain to the peripheral part of the body and 80% of afferent fibers with an opposite function where the signals from the "periphery" arrive at the "central site" or the brain. Vagus nerve stimulation is a topic that needs to be further explored, however a mediation of the vagus nerve on depressive, inflammatory, metabolic altered states and heart failure is very likely. Just think that it was observed as early as 1880, yes you understood correctly. 1800, that manual massage and compression of the carotid artery of the cervical region could prevent epileptic attacks (Lanska, 2002). Only in the middle of the last century, between the thirties and forties, the stimulation with electrical equipment was tried to understand interactions with brain activity. Cardio-respiratory stimulation of the vagus nerve can explain the many emotional and cognitive benefits that can be obtained thanks to deep breathing, yoga, or aerobic activities and exercises. In fact, the vagus nerve has a direct and indirect connection with the cortical, limbic, thalamus, and striatal neurological circuits involved in the relevant cognitive and emotional functions in cases of depression (Ruffoli et al., 2011).

Pros and Cons: Possible Negative Effects

Some negative repercussions may also exist here and are related only to the moment of stimulation, so only for a limited period of time that can happen if you stimulate any other part of your body. Remember that 80% of the fibers of the vagus nerve are afferent so they send the signal to the brain, where you will feel pain, not so much in the affected part of the body. By stimulating the left side of the nerve (present at the middle cervical) you may notice an alteration in the tone of the voice, cough, breathlessness (dyspnea), difficulty in swallowing (dysphagia), pain in the neck, or an alteration in the sensitivity of the limbs (paraesthesia) such as tingling. The left vagus nerve is believed to have the ability to minimize any cardiac effects such as bradycardia (irregular or slow heartbeat) or asystole (absence of cardiac systole that blocks circulation and is fatal in a very short time if the person is not resuscitated) which are generally controlled by the right vagus nerve.

Headache, Migraine, or Cluster Headache?

I guess you will know these terms not only from hearsay but because you suffered from these pains at work or while sleeping and maybe it improved a little only during the day. Well, then you are in the right place because in this and the next sections we will talk about that. The BOE (Britannica Online Encyclopedia) defines headache as a widespread pain in the head area that varies in intensity and severity based on the cause. 10% of people suffer from recurring **headaches**. Many episodes arise from parts of the skull or very pain-sensitive neighboring points that are damaged or over-stimulated. Some of these structures are intracranial, or tissues that surround or are located outside the skull. When you drink too much and you get a headache, in that case, the headache occurs inside the skull and is due to a temporary increase in blood supply; however, it can also be a consequence of, for example, fever or a sudden increase in blood pressure. Conversely, examples of extracranial headaches can be caused by dilation of the arteries present outside the skull that supply superficial tissues or support the musculoskeletal structures of the face, neck, and scalp. Excessive tiredness, tension, neck and eye strain can all cause headaches of this type. 90% of tension headaches are precisely caused by the distension of the extracranial artery or to support the contraction of the neck muscles rather than the facial muscles, due to fatigue, stress, frustration, or depression. You will be realizing how everything is connected and what impact it has on your daily life and how you deal with it, whether it is positive or negative.

Migraine, the BOE article continues, is often accompanied by nausea and vomiting, you can suffer from it every day as once a year but in most cases, it occurs once or twice a month. Often a migraine attack is triggered by an external stimulus such as a particularly stressful situation, a hormonal change such as can occur during the menstrual cycle, the intake of certain foods or beverages that are not necessarily alcoholic. Only a few people experience symptoms such as numbness, dizziness, loss of vision, or temporary defects in speech or movements that just precede the actual migraine. Unfortunately, movements, direct and very intense lights, and physical activity tend to make the pain worse. Some curiosities:

- The underlying cause of migraine remains uncertain, perhaps it could be hereditary since between 75–90% of those who suffer from it report a family history of this problem.
- Almost 2/3 of the people who suffer from it are women.
- Migraines often occur with a high frequency in people who are particularly workaholics and who impose very high standards on themselves, increasing the stress they undergo.
- Migraines could be caused by an abnormality in the regulation of serotonin used by the body to send impulses to the brain.

Based on the identification of the factor that most activates and triggers the migraine attack, it will then be easier to understand which drug or other remedies may be more suitable for preventing it.

Cluster headache, on the other hand, is characterized by sudden pain in the area surrounding the eye or in a part of the face. It is often accompanied by tearing and watery eyes, sweating, or a stuffy nose. The pain usually does not persist for more than two hours but has a high frequency which can be daily, weekly or monthly; two triggers can be stress or alcohol consumption. A curiosity:

- In this case, men are affected more than women and usually, the most affected age group is a very wide range between 20 and 60 years.

Smartphone Syndrome: Effect on the "Text Neck" Musculature

We have briefly mentioned it in the previous sections, but it deserves further attention given the frequency with which the head is tilted forward during the hours spent in front of the PC for work or in front of the smartphone during breaks.

The habit of holding this position forward considerably increases the weight to be supported for many muscle groups present in the cervical spine whose task is precisely to support the head (Morrison, 2018).

Over time, this position can lead to muscle imbalance as the body attempts to adapt to both continue to support the head and to find an efficient way to facilitate the sight of nearby objects. Part of the muscles thus becomes weak and elongated, while other muscle groups shorten and stiffen.

Muscle Bands That Stretch and Weaken

- **Deep cervical flexors:** Also called the long head muscles, they are located in the front of the cervical spine and help stabilize the neck (splenius, Figure 4). When they weaken, they lengthen as the chin moves away from the neck, which is known as a protruding chin.

- **Erector spine muscle:** It belongs to the muscular fascia of the vertebral arches and extends throughout the spine. In this case, we refer to the part between the end of the cervical tract and the beginning of the chest. This muscle plays a key role in the rotation and lengthening of the spine and, as it stretches and loses strength, it is no longer able to keep the neck and upper back lifted and prevent them from bending forward.

- **Shoulder blade retractor muscle:** The middle trapezius (Trapezius) and the rhomboid muscle (Rhomboides) of the upper back help keep the shoulder blades back. Do you know when we say belly in and chest out?! Here, you succeed thanks to these two muscles! When the shoulder blades are weakened, they are able to rotate forward more easily thus contributing to poor posture.

For this reason, as we will also see later, these muscle groups can be the subject of targeted exercises that strengthen them. By strengthening the muscles and above all understanding the importance of this remedy, you will have a double benefit: correcting this wrong position and relieving neck pain. Figure 4 helps you understand where these muscle groups are located:

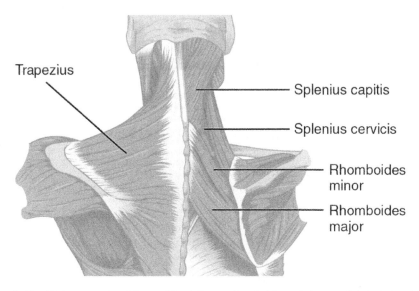

Figure 3: Simplified representation of the muscle bands between the end of the cervical tract and the beginning of the thorax. [4]

Muscle Bands That Shorten and Stiffen

- **Suboccipital muscles (Figure 5):** There are 4 pairs of small muscle bands that connect the back of the skull to the beginning of the cervical spine and also contribute to rotation and extension movements. They are muscle bands that work incessantly to allow you to keep your head up and look straight ahead when keeping a straight posture.

- **Bibs:** As the upper back muscles tend to stretch and the shoulders curve forward, the chest muscles tend to shorten and stiffen. The

[4] Source Figure 4:
https://commons.wikimedia.org/wiki/File:1117_Muscles_of_the_Neck_Upper_Back.png
Credits: OpenStax College, CC BY 3.0 <https://creativecommons.org/licenses/by/3.0>, via Wikimedia Commons

same applies to the minor pectorals located in the upper part of the chest and have a triangular shape.

- **Levator scapula muscle (Figure 5):** Located along the back and laterally to the neck, it reaches the shoulder blade. The Levator muscle plays a fundamental role in the ability to lift and rotate the scapula and shoulder and, by holding incorrect positions, it is a muscle that can contract.

This musculature is also at the center of attention for targeted exercises.

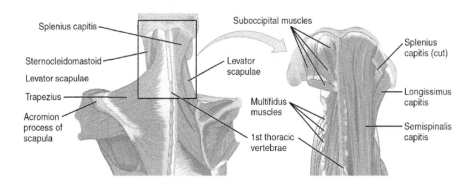

Figure 4: Overview of the cervical muscles subject to contractions. [5]

5   Source   Figure   5:
https://commons.wikimedia.org/wiki/File:1111_Posterior_and_Side_Views_of_the_Neck_b_an
d_c.png Credits: OpenStax College, CC BY 3.0 <https://creativecommons.org/licenses/by/3.0>,
via Wikimedia Commons

Symptoms of Smartphone Syndrome

Morrison (2018), concludes this interesting overview of the musculature affected by this problem by briefly mentioning some symptoms:

- **General inflammation and soreness:** Which spreads through the upper back, neck, head, and shoulders.

- **Intense and localized pain:** When a muscle is tense or has spasms, it can cause pain that can be perceived as sharp or with a sharp burning sensation that can get worse with a certain position or by making a certain movement or vice versa it can improve.

- **Pain trigger points:** Specific points that become even more painful when stressed. Some studies have linked these particularly sensitive points on the head, shoulders, and neck as being present mainly in people suffering from migraines and headaches.

- **Muscle stiffness:** When too stressed, the muscles stiffen easily or respond in this way when there is further inflammation in the surrounding areas such as the presence of a hernia. As a result, the cervical spine becomes much more rigid, and the range of motion is reduced.

This incorrect posture can then lead to pain in the joints, discs, nerve roots, and other elements present on site.

Part 2

Vertigo and Dizziness

Drowsiness, lightheadedness, dizziness, and then neck pains break out; sometimes, when you're lucky, you can anticipate the pain a little and manage it enough with an anti-inflammatory, right? Now you will understand more about the cause of this malaise. Although it is still under study, several factors affect it, often the result of an atlanto-occipital misalignment between the head and the neck, a whiplash, the dissection of some arteries (Gross, 2018). In the latter case, the sensation of dizziness derives from the interruption of blood circulation in the inner ear or the brain stem. Arthritis, surgery, and trauma are all events that can lead to cervical vertigo. The muscles and joints of the neck are composed of receptors that send signals to the brain about the movements you make with the head and the vestibular apparatus, located in the inner ear, is responsible for balance and acts in synergy with other parts of the body to maintain muscle coordination as well. When this mechanism does not work as it should, the receptors fail to transmit signals to the brain and cause lightheadedness and other sensory dysfunctions. Arthritis was mentioned as a cause a little while ago; in the hypothesis of cervical spondylosis (a chronic disorder caused by wear and degeneration of the joints), this can lead to increased pressure on the spinal cord and/or spinal nerves and hinder blood flow to the brain and inner ear. Even a simple hernia without degenerative conditions of this type can lead to the same problem. In Nguyen (2019) two other rare possible causes are added:

- **Bow hunter syndrome:** That is, in rare cases, lateral rotation of the head can compress the vertebral artery causing a sensation of spinning in some people. This syndrome is more likely to affect the C1-C2 vertebrae such as a misalignment of these vertebrae or other spinal abnormalities.

- **Myofascial cervical headache syndrome:** Also not very common, it affects the neck muscles and connective tissue. Its cause is unknown, but it is estimated that 30% of people who suffer from it also have dizziness and dizziness among the symptoms. This condition is usually treated with specific physiotherapy, drugs, or local injections.

In some cases, pain in the cervical tract and dizziness may have origins outside the anatomical part itself. Among these we find stress and anxiety that lead to sensations of dizziness and a feeling of light-headedness and Ménière's disease, a pathology of the inner ear whose cause is still unknown, and which can include a coming and going of symptoms such as dizziness, problems with hearing and tinnitus when perceiving sounds in higher pitches, buzzing or other disturbances even in the absence of external noises (Nguyen, 2019). Overall, the sensations that are experienced can be enclosed in the following: general inflammation and soreness from the skull to the shoulders, an acute even intermittent pain that can extend to the hand and arm, a feeling of staggering, fainting or sudden drowsiness, the pressure felt in one or both ears, visual changes and increased sensitivity in the limbs involved which worsens by locally increasing pressure. Some activities can make the situation even worse such as lateral movement of the head, sports such as running or weightlifting, or other sports that involve sudden jerky movements.

Diagnosis

There is no precise test to be carried out to identify cervical dizziness immediately, this diagnosis is often reached by exclusion (Reiley et al., 2017), for this reason, a complete medical history of the patient is necessary as the symptoms are common to multiple pathologies, in this case, to be excluded, such as heart problems, drug intake and particular neurological conditions.

The Polyvagal Theory

In this sub-chapter, you will learn more about the polyvagal theory, useful for understanding the impact that traumas of different nature have on your nervous system. This theory, studied by neurophysiologist Stephen Porges (2014) aims to explain the reactions that occur in dangerous situations as the defensive system that your body activates, in this case, does not start from the cortical areas but from the brainstem which represents the oldest part of the brain (State of Mind Magazine, 2021). The article in this magazine continues by citing a fundamental distinction to keep in mind: first of all, you must understand the underlying difference between reptilian and mammalian ancestors. Mammals (us) need social relationships, to defend each other and to create emotional bonds; on the contrary, reptiles are solitary animals. It follows that in the evolutionary path the nervous system of both has had different evolutions to allow the survival of the species. There are two fundamental branches of the autonomic nervous system: the first concerns the attack-flight and freezing reactions that are activated in conditions of medium danger through the sympathetic system; the second, using the dorsal-vagal (parasympathetic) system triggers what is called apparent death. In the case of mammals, a third branch developed which was active only in conditions of sufficient safety, namely the ventral-vagal parasympathetic system which concerns the behaviors of mutual aid, collaboration, and attachment. Usually, this third branch goes a little into the background and there is a tendency to favor a more classical view that contrasts the sympathetic system (attack-flight) to the parasympathetic (vagal, responsible for the decrease of arousal, i.e., a state where the body assumes a very high vigilance and is ready to react when needed). In the article, we ask ourselves if hyperactivity is our only defense and, the first difference that distinguishes this classic vision from the polyvagal theory, is to always keep in mind that the response to the challenges that the environment in which we live sends us derives precisely from our evolutionary history. The autonomic nervous system works on hierarchical levels; that is, to protect us, it first exploits the adaptive responses of the most recent evolutionary stages, and gradually, when these are not sufficient, it relies on the most ancient evolutionary stages. In the course of evolution, we find two different branches of the parasympathetic system:

1. **The most recent vagal circuit (ventral-vagal)**: Is composed of afferent fibers (remember that they are the fibers that carry impulses from the periphery of the body to the brain) that affect the organs above the diaphragm, that is: the muscles of the face and the ability to express emotions using facial expressions, pharynx, heart, lungs, breath, and voice. In dangerous situations, this circuit allows to calm the heart and stimulates social activities.

2. **The oldest vagal circuit (dorsal-vagal):** This affects the organs underlying the diaphragm such as the stomach, small intestine, bladder, and colon, and which plays a very important role in maintaining homeostasis and the functioning visceral functions of the organs just mentioned. In this case, however, in situations of danger, this circuit promotes a response that we have inherited from reptiles, namely the collapse that nowadays in humans can also be lethal or depending on the situation it also leads to fainting.

48

Polyvagal Theory and Vagus Nerve

This theory, therefore, places emphasis on the existence of these two circuits, on the importance of the various evolutionary phases as sources of resources on which to draw and consider defense responses as adaptations to the challenges of the surrounding environment. The concept on which we want to emphasize is how much the autonomic nervous system is constantly engaged in defensive actions including traumatic situations or prolonged stress. Without going very far, you can find these episodes in your daily life; when you find yourself carrying out tasks that require a very high attention span, or with situations and people that are emotionally difficult to manage. All this affects your mental and physical well-being because the balance between the different branches of the nervous system is lost. The name "polyvagal" theory originates from the fact that the Vagus Nerve is made up of a family of nerves. Let's be clear. As mentioned before, you have seen that there are two vagal circuits: the ventral-vagal (more recent) and dorsal-vagal (older) composed of many nerve endings, and each circuit is involved in the management of certain organs and movements whose lowest common denominator is to be an active part in the social interactions of which we mammals are oriented.

The Most Archaic Circuit: Dorsal-Vagal

A few more concepts to better understand how it helps us every day: it is activated when we are in serious danger and simulates an apparent death by slowing down our functions (typical defense strategy of reptiles).

However, the basis of this "freezing" is based on an extreme state of fear and, in higher mammals, this is linked to loss of control, mental clouding, and emotions such as disgust, sadness, and a sense of embarrassment, as well as fear. You know when your gaze is lost in the void, soft muscles, a tired and heavy body, you retract your neck back, your heartbeat slows down?! On these occasions, the dorsal-vagal circuit is activated. It is frequently associated with depressive conditions, there is a decrease in oxygen supply, and a slowdown in musculoskeletal responses. Over time, evolution has led to the development of the sympathetic system that regulates metabolic capacity, heartbeat, and other physiological reactions related to this fight-flight response that are activated in dangerous conditions. At the base, there are always emotions such as anger and fear, when the sympathetic system is activated you return to have better oxygenation, an increase in a heartbeat; in short, a substantial increase in mobilization.

The Next Evolution: The Ventral-Vagal Circuit

This circuit is specific for higher mammals and for humans. Also in this case it has a calming and slowing down effect of various functions, but the difference lies in the fact that there are no emotions of fear and there are no dangerous situations. In this case, the movements are more harmonious, there is no muscle stiffening as in the previous situation, there is a modulation of the middle ear muscles which improves the ability to listen and understand. So it is interesting to note how from a very primitive and archaic system, this has gone to refine over time becoming more and more sophisticated and trained to quickly activate or deactivate some circuits when passing from a safety situation (ventral-vagal) to a dangerous situation (sympathetic system).

Polyvagal Syndrome Cluster

The article continues by citing how Stephen Porges tried to identify four clusters, situations that serve to outline a progression of symptoms and responses within the individual:

1. The first context that is indicated is the moment in which there is an attenuation of social interaction which also leads to a decrease in ventral vagal activity. This manifests itself in the upper part of the orbicular muscles, high sensitivity to sounds, and an overall low reactivity.

2. The second context identified considers a high reactivity and mobilization directly connected with the sympathetic system. In this case, there is a rapid shift between states of anxiety and hypervigilance to an emotional state of calm.

3. The third cluster alternates between the sympathetic and dorsal-vagal systems. Alternation that manifests itself with intestinal problems, fibromyalgia, hypotension, and reduced mobilization.

4. The last situation is the actual dissociation with a chronic collapse resulting from dorsal-vagal activation resulting from a situation of danger or stress. Unfortunately, it occurs very frequently in people who are victims of abuse and violence.

Polyvagal Theory and Trauma

How do traumatic situations affect physiology? The article goes on to explain that when relationships and social connections are less, negative effects also occur at the body level. In communication, there are some elements that act on the myelinated (ventral-vagal) vagal nerve which controls the activation of defense reactions. We are talking about intonation, emotional contents, and prosody (linguistic cadence). When you perceive social situations of danger, reciprocity in communication and connection to the other person is lost. These emotionally complex and unpleasant episodes are the cause in the brain of the violation of "a neural expectation" given by reciprocity as we said before. If you have experienced trauma, you will probably be inclined to take a conservative attitude where even neutral situations will be more likely to be considered dangerous. Without going into the details of clinical experiences, it is interesting to mention a further statement in the article: traumatizing experiences such as aggressions, catastrophes, or any other experience tend to remain etched in our memory precisely because the activation of the dorsal-vagal system is, for the human body, comparable in all respects to a mortal experience and therefore from this we understand the important therapeutic implications that such studies have in helping people to re-elaborate these experiences and consider them in a different perspective. Some practices have a positive effect and allow you to activate the ventral-vagal circuit which, in situations perceived as safe, helps to promote a feeling of further safety. These are:

- **Breathing.** Inhaling slowly but exhaling for a long time (avoiding hyperventilation), singing since it is an activity that leads to prolonged breathing, and choral singing that requires tuning in with others, high-frequency music.

- **Cardiac coherence exercises always with long breaths**. All this to try to evoke positive experiences and to be more familiar with the states of regulation.

Part 3

11 Techniques to Control Chronic Pain

To fully understand how to deal with chronic pain, it is useful to understand how to derive the maximum benefit from concentration and breathing techniques in order to relax the body. It may seem easy to relax but it is not always like that, it requires a little practice but it is worth the effort to focus no longer on pain and being able to relax the muscles and the tension accumulated throughout the body. Several factors come into play when you feel chronic pain, you can consider it as a matryoshka, Figure 6 below helps you to schematize the concept:

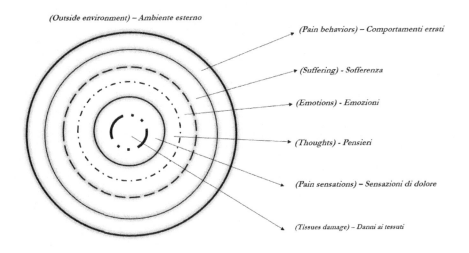

(Outside environment) – Ambiente esterno

(Pain behaviors) – Comportamenti errati

(Suffering) - Sofferenza

(Emotions) - Emozioni

(Thoughts) - Pensieri

(Pain sensations) – Sensazioni di dolore

(Tissues damage) – Danni ai tessuti

Figure 5: Levels of chronic pain interaction. [6]

[6] Copyright Figure 6: Emma Gentile. Recreated from scratch from the page https://www.spine-health.com/conditions/chronic-pain/understanding-chronic-pain

As indicated by Deardorff (2017) in Figure 6, there are various levels of chronic pain interaction. Starting from the innermost part of your body or the **lesions** to the tissues that are the origin of the pain itself as they transmit the pain signal to the nervous system. At the second level, we find the **sensation** of pain that the brain actually perceives after sending the signal from the periphery to the central nervous system. **Thoughts**, like the events around you, have a great influence both consciously and unconsciously on how pain is perceived; just think of the positive fatigue accused after an hour of sport, rather than the negative fatigue that derives from a pathology. **Emotions** are your personal response deriving from the thoughts you have about the pain you are feeling, therefore your way of dealing with it. If it comes from a very serious condition your emotional response will tend to consider fear, anxiety, or depression for example. The word **suffering** is distinct from the term pain, although they are sometimes used interchangeably, however it is also closely linked to the emotional aspect of pain.

Now let's get to the heart of the 11 techniques that help us to better manage chronic pain. First of all, it is important to check your breathing by preparing a quiet space that invites you to relax, a dimly lit or dark room depending on your preferences, take a lying position and start with deep breaths using the chest to breathe and not the abdomen for a few minutes. These eleven techniques use visualization to relieve pain (Block, 2007):

1. **Shift the focus:** This technique is considered very powerful because it demonstrates the ability of the mind to change the sensations the body feels. An example is to take attention away

from the painful point and focus on a point of your body that does not present any problems. For example: imagining that your hands are warming helps you to divert attention from the pain you feel in a different part of the body.

2. **Dissociation:** As the name already indicates, there is a tendency to mentally separate the painful part from the rest of the body; you can also imagine the mind and body as two separate entities thus removing the pain you feel from the rest of the body. An example: if you have back pain try to imagine the painful part of the back sitting in a chair on the opposite side of the room you are in and order it to stay there, a mental representation that keeps it away from where you are.

3. **Stratifying the sensations:** If, for example, a pain produces a sensation of heat: separate the sensation of heat from that of pain.

4. **Mental anesthesia:** It means imagining that you are injected with a painkiller, or that dry ice or other remedies are placed on the painful part and think about the feelings of cooling and well-being that these entail.

5. **Analgesic effect:** Along the lines of the previous one.

6. **Hand transfer:** In this case, as in the previous ones, you imagine a better condition, opposite to the painful one you are experiencing, and helping yourself with your hand, to make it more concrete, you place it on top of the part.

7. **Progression/regression of age:** Projecting oneself into the past or the future in a situation of absence of pain or very limited pain and visualizing it as if it were the present moment.

8. **Symbolic visualization:** Imagine something symbolic that indicates chronic pain such as very strong lights or a boring noise. Gradually reduce the annoying characteristics you have attributed to this symbol; for example, decrease the volume or decrease the intensity of the light and thus decrease the pain itself.

9. **Positive visualization:** Shift your focus on something you like, on your favorite vacation, the sea, the mountains, where you feel good and relax more easily.

10. **Counting:** It may seem trivial, but counting your breaths, some objects you find yourself observing, or anything else like tiles, helps to distract your mind.

11. **Painful movements:** Mentally try to visualize the pain you have in an area of your body where you can bear it more easily.

They seem simple but you can learn some of these techniques best with the help of an expert and it takes a little patience and practice to be able to apply them to the fullest. Block (2007) suggests practicing for about 30 minutes three times a week; being able to relax and master these techniques can help to have long-term benefits and can be put into practice even while doing other activities.

Progressive Muscle Relaxation

The goal to be achieved is to relieve tension and restore psychophysiological balance; in the light of what you have learned so far, knowing a relaxation technique will certainly be an additional means at your disposal to better experience some situations. Specifically, this technique was proposed at the beginning of the last century by Edmund Jacobson and is based on the idea that a person's emotional state and thoughts affect the level of muscular response by emphasizing the interaction between thought, muscles, and emotions (Jacobson, 1929). In this article on the website "studicognitiva.it" (see bibliography), this technique is described as extremely useful not only for those suffering from insomnia or other disorders related to rest but also for those who need to manage aggression more effectively, daily stress, and anger. First of all, the first thing you need to do if you want to try this method is to develop the ability to identify and distinguish the state of muscle tension, doing specific exercises to increase awareness and feel even the slightest muscle contractions. Once you get used to it you will be able to relax the muscles not interested in a specific movement thus using only the necessary muscle tension. The central point of this technique consists in alternating, following well-defined timing, states of tension, and relaxation of certain parts of the body. According to Jacobson's observations, noticing the feeling of relaxation when you stop contracting the muscles will allow the person to experience a pleasant sensation that will result in psychological well-being. Specifically, it is also beneficial in situations of very high general tension that exacerbates somatic problems (migraines, vomiting attacks, somatizations), anxiety, phobias and mood disorders, management of high stress in the family, at work, or in the financial sector. It is a useful technique as a support for dealing with important situations such as public speaking or sports competitions. This technique is accompanied by the much more common **autogenic training** or self-induced exercises that induce pleasant visualizations.

Lower and Upper Relaxation Exercises

The article concludes by making a distinction between **lower** and **higher** relaxation exercises. In the lower type exercises, the focus is on body sensations, while in the second type the focus is placed on mental visualization. There are six different exercises, the first two are defined as fundamental while the remaining complementary:

1. Exercise of the heaviness that acts on the relaxation of the muscles.
2. Exercise of heat, which affects the peripheral blood vessels and their dilation.
3. Exercise of the heart that affects cardiac function.
4. Exercise of the solar plexus which acts on the organs of the abdomen.
5. A breathing exercise that affects the respiratory system.
6. The exercise of the cool forehead instead acts on the brain.

Meditation: 11 Scientifically Proven Benefits

Being able to start this practice is not always obvious for everyone, for some it is very intuitive, others may find it difficult to slow down the frenetic pace they are used to every day, relax and carve out even a few minutes for themselves. Sometimes it is thought that to meditate you need to carve out hours of time, in reality starting with five to ten minutes is enough. Now we see 11 benefits or eleven situations in which meditating helps to increase your psychophysical well-being and reduce the states of tension that accumulate in the muscle groups and that can be reflected in the cervical and vagus nerve problems we are treating. Thorpe (2020) cites, among the reasons why meditation is increasingly widespread, the ability to increase discipline, the quality of sleep, and the pain threshold. Let's see why meditation is mostly used for:

1. **Stress reduction:** This is the main reason why people choose this practice. A study conducted by a pool of scientists (Goyal et al., 2014) has actually confirmed how it is able to reduce the state of stress, usually due to very high levels of cortisol. In fact, this hormone contributes to the negative effects of stress such as the release of cytokines, inflammatory chemical compounds. This can affect sleep quality, increased blood pressure, anxiety and depression, lack of mental clarity, and fatigue. Mindfulness meditation in particular contributed significantly to a decrease in stress in an eight-week study (Rosenkranz et al., 2013). Other observed benefits relate to irritable bowel syndrome (Cearley et al.,

2017), fibromyalgia (Aman et al., 2018), and post-traumatic stress disorder (Hilton et al., 2017).

2. **Promotes mental health:** A subject that tends to be underestimated and not talked about enough, it helps to promote a more conscious and positive image of oneself. An interesting study (Kiken and Shook, 2014) actually showed how a group of people encouraged a positive mental approach after doing a meditation exercise. Do you remember we mentioned cytokines earlier? Here, it seems that the levels of these chemical compounds are decreasing.

3. **Increase self-awareness:** Some forms of meditation that place reflection on personal questions at the center of the practice, encourage the person to improve, get to know each other better, and grow. Other practices prompt you to recognize thoughts and habits that can be harmful or disempowering so that you can improve. The development of a creative and problem-solving approach is not to be underestimated.

4. **Increase the attention span:** Meditative practices that focus precisely on attention can be concentrated for longer periods and perform better at work or when required. Furthermore, another study concluded that meditation can even subvert the brain's tendency to wander the mind, worry, and get distracted easily (Sood and Jones, 2013).

5. **It can help reduce memory loss due to age:** Among the positive effects of meditation, there is an increase in attention and reflexes, and clarity of thought that benefit the mind and keep it more

reactive. Kirtan Kriya is a meditative practice that combines chants or mantras with a repetitive movement of the fingers aimed at focusing your thoughts; this method has been seen to be useful and beneficial in those suffering from age-related memory loss.

6. **Help people be kinder:** Some practices encourage a positive attitude towards self-respect and respect for others. Metta is an example of a practice that begins by creating kind thoughts about yourself. With practice, people are able to develop compassion and kindness to project them outside towards friends, acquaintances, and finally towards people with whom we are less in tune, creating greater understanding and interpersonal interactions.

7. **It can help fight addictions:** By helping you to develop self-discipline and redirect the focus of your attention by increasing awareness and control of yourself, it allows you to use these tools to more easily manage addictions, including the uncontrolled desire for food.

8. **Improves the night's rest:** Unfortunately almost half of the population happens sooner or later to suffer from insomnia. A comparative study (Ong et al., 2014) noted that those who meditate regularly remain asleep longer, managing to get rid of the tension accumulated in the body, calming down, and falling asleep earlier.

9. **Helps to control chronic pain:** The perception of pain is directly linked to your mood and leads, as mentioned several times so far, to very high levels of stress. Thanks to the practice and techniques you have learned it will be easier for you to manage it.

10. **It can help you lower blood pressure:** In some cases, conditions of prolonged exertion and very high blood pressure can contribute to different diseases over the years. Thanks to meditation, it is possible to relax the signals that coordinate cardiac activity and the state of alertness that is triggered in certain situations (Olex et al., 2013).

11. **Where you want, when you want:** You don't need a particular space or equipment, you only need a few minutes a day to get started.

One piece of advice that Thorpe (2020) gives is to choose the type of meditation you prefer based on the goal you want to achieve. There are two main styles of meditation:

- The first focuses on a single object, thought, sound or visualization in such a way as to eliminate distractions from your mind through breathing, relaxing sounds, or mantras.
- The second type considers the environment as a whole, trains the thinking and perception of yourself. It invites you to become more aware of long-buried impulses, sensations, or feelings.

Consider carving out even five minutes just for you in the morning and get started easily thanks to apps, free classes, courses, or the online resources you prefer.

Vagus Nerve: How to Stimulate It

As you have already seen in part in the section of the polyvagal theory, the vagus nerve works by counterbalancing the attack and flight modality of the nervous system and represents a truly powerful source of energy and well-being. It is therefore worthwhile to understand how to best stimulate it since it works a bit like the reset button.

The Vagal Tone

Vagal tone, or the activity of the vagus nerve, is important in activating the parasympathetic nervous system and is mainly measured by observing the heart rate. Accelerate briefly when you inhale and slow down a little while exhaling. The greater the difference between inhalation and exhalation, the higher we consider the vagal tone. The higher the vagal tone, the more you will be able to relax. The presence of a very high vagal tone is associated with the greater well-being of the person; it helps you in regulating blood sugar, reduces the risk of heart attack and cardiovascular disease, reduces migraines, and improves your digestion. I would like to point out that also from this point of view meditation, deep breathing exercises and other techniques that we will see shortly are useful for activating the Vagus Nerve and consequently, decreasing both emotional and physical stress and also to better manage neck pain. Elevated vagal tone is also associated with greater emotional stability, longevity, and resilience. On the contrary, low vagal tone is associated with mood swings, depression, diabetes, chronic inflammation, chronic fatigue syndrome and possible sleep disorders, cardiovascular diseases, and cognitive deficits. By stimulating the Vagus Nerve you will also stimulate the parasympathetic nervous system which in turn will reduce your neurophysiological response to stress, reduce your heart rate, affect both the limbic system of the brain where your emotions are processed and the digestive system creating a feeling of well-being. In general, it helps you to better manage the feeling of discomfort you feel when you are under stress, tension (which also spills over into different muscle groups), anxiety, and depression (Innis, Accessed: June 2021).

Methods for Activating the Vagus Nerve

There are really quite a few of them and we will distinguish between those that find greater accuracy and scientific evidence and some methods that may be useful but do not yet find solid confirmation. I remind you to rely on your doctor or specialist and not to improvise these methods, even more, if you find yourself living with heavy situations of panic attacks, anxiety, or depression. An initial piece of advice is to listen and increase awareness of how your body reacts to stress or other demanding situations, so as to recognize the signals and be able to help it in the best way. The methodologies reported are taken from Cohen et al. (2021).

Cold Exposure

According to some studies, when the human body adapts to colder temperatures, the sympathetic nervous system responsible for the fight-flight response is lowered, favoring the resting system of the parasympathetic system which is mediated by the Vagus Nerve. This study considers as cold temperatures around 10°C (50°F), sudden exposure of up to 4°C (39°F) activates the vagus nerve even more. Without going to particular places, many people prefer to take cold showers and in some cultures such as the Nordic countries, exposure to the cold is also present in holidays celebrated with swimming in the ocean in winter or early spring.

Singing

Well yes! Even if you are out of tune and have always preferred to avoid, you should know that singing increases heart rate variability, allows you to relax, and develop better resilience and adaptation to stress by activating parasympathetic activity. The study conducted by Vickhoff et al. (2013) noted how chanting and murmuring mantras, hymns, or music of a certain rhythm are activities that, even when carried out in a group, send relaxing inputs to the brain and activate both the vagus nerve and the sympathetic nervous system so as to allow people to reach a state of flow. Religious choral songs are also an excellent example of this. An extensive bibliography is not available for this particular aspect, however, the social interactions that allow you to solidify this activity rather than the passion and energy that a person puts into it certainly helps to detach the mind from the day's commitments.

Yoga and Meditation

Some studies indicate an increase in parasympathetic activity thanks to yoga. The benefits of this activity associated with an improvement in

66

anxiety states and the overall well-being of the person are known. However, further research is needed to understand the specific effect on vagal tone. We have dedicated an entire section to the benefits of meditation and it is interesting to underline how this activity can indirectly stimulate the Vagus Nerve. Nevertheless, deep breathing exercises are very effective, focusing only on the breath that stimulates the ventral-vagal system, since the Vagus Nerve passes right through the anatomical tract of the vocal cords.

A Positive Approach and Social Interactions

A positive approach does not mean pretending that everything is fine even when the world is collapsing on you, this is just a counterproductive mask and on a subconscious level you know it is not. A positive approach, in this case, refers to adopting and developing a capacity for gratitude towards life and every time the mind begins to wander it returns to repeating affirmations such as "may you feel protected, may you feel safe and happy." In one study they showed how, by increasing joy, serenity, or hope, the sense of connection with other people also expanded, and an improvement in vagal activity indicated by the variability of heart rate (Kok et al., 2013).

Slow and Deep Breathing

This type of breathing is very common in meditation techniques, yoga, and relaxation techniques as mentioned several times. Your heart and cervical spine contain types of neurons called baroreceptors. Baroreceptors are specialized neurons that recognize blood pressure and transmit the signal to the brain. When you have high blood pressure, the signal helps to activate the vagus nerve which in turn will communicate with the heart to decrease blood pressure and heartbeat. This will limit the sympathetic system's fight-and-flight response and make it easier for you to relax. The sensitivity of the baroreceptors varies considerably and, if too sensitive, this mechanism is triggered very easily. According to the study by Mason et al. (2013) who tested the effects of slow yogic breathing called *ujjayi*, an increase in the sensitivity of baroreceptors and vagal activity was seen, thus managing to decrease blood pressure. This type of breathing consists of six breaths per minute, taking five seconds to inhale and as many seconds to exhale. Some researchers claim that it helps manage and reduce anxiety, however, this is not yet confirmed. In the practice of yoga, it is emphasized that breathing should be slow and start from the belly, and the more it expands, the deeper the breathing is.

Smiling Is the Best Medicine

Not only popular wisdom but also interesting scientific results underline its benefits (Miller and Fry, 2009). There are still many aspects being studied to understand the specific relationship between laughter and the activation of the vagus nerve, and some researchers in particular are investigating the beneficial effects that laughter can have on cognitive functions and protection from cardiovascular disease. Some research has indicated that laughter increases the level of beta-endorphins and nitrogen monoxide to benefit the vascular system. (Miller e Fry, 2009).

Praying

When praying, the activity of the cardiovascular rhythm is strengthened by reducing the diastolic blood pressure and increasing the variability of heart rate, an indication of a higher vagal tone. Keep in mind that the recitation of prayers or mantras is accompanied by deeper breathing with the relative benefits that we talked about earlier. (Bernardi et al., 2001).

Magnetotherapy and Lying Down on the Right Side

Some scientists hypothesize that this type of therapy is useful for stimulating the vagus nerve as it increases cardiac variability, however further studies are needed to have more confirmations also regarding the best position for bedtime. In fact, it is assumed that lying down on the right side stimulates vagal activity more, which instead decreases by remaining lying on the back.

Use of Probiotics and Intermittent Fasting

As you have previously learned, there is a close relationship between the vagus nerve, the digestive system, and impulses that are sent to the brain, and it is more and more evident the importance that the intestinal flora covers, so much that it is defined as a gut-brain axis. In a study conducted on mice, providing them with the probiotic Lactobacillus rhamnosus, a positive alteration of GABA receptors, one of the most important types of the central nervous system, which among other functions also regulate mood, was seen (Bravo et al., 2011). Intermittent fasting and reduced calorie intake seem to increase vagal tone, but further studies need to be conducted for more confirmation. The hypothesis behind it is that the vagus nerve can mediate a lowering of metabolism and blood glucose level during fasting, thus reducing chemical signals. On the contrary, the satiety stimulus that comes after meals could increase sympathetic activity.

Exercise, Massage, and Tai Chi

Not very intense sporting activity and the massage of some areas such as the carotid artery can stimulate the vagus nerve. Some research indicates that massage (performed by a professional) can help reduce seizures (Green and Weaver, 2014). Other studies have found that pressure massage in children allowed them to gain weight, another function mediated mainly by the vagus nerve. Equally useful for stimulating the vagus is also given by a foot reflexology massage and the practice of Thai Chi.

Omega 3, Omega 6, Zinc, and Fiber

An increase in vagal activity is attributed to the intake of EPA (omega 3, anti-inflammatory fatty acids that you can find in fish for example) and DHA (omega 6, which on the contrary stimulate inflammation). Some scientists believe that this is precisely why omega 3s are considered very important for the heart (Von Schacky, 2006). Zinc also seems to be beneficial; it is a very common mineral, but it is often underestimated. Fiber intake is also considered likely to stimulate the development of the satiety hormone called GLP-1 which in turn stimulates vagal impulses to the brain.

Experimental Stimulation Methods

While the previous methods are accompanied by scientific evidence, the approaches mentioned below need further investigation:

- **Gargle:** The Vagus Nerve flows in the back of the throat muscles allowing you to gargle, during which, in theory, you would be able to contract this muscle which could activate vagal activity and stimulate gastrointestinal activity.

- **Use of a tongue depressor:** Thanks to this tool you stimulate the pharyngeal reflex of vomiting, a reflex directly linked to the back muscles of the throat where the vagus passes.

- **Coughing and tension in the stomach muscles.**

- **Enemas.**

- **Insulin.**

- **Ginger:** It is hypothesized that ginger can prevent nausea and vomiting by inhibiting the function of the vagus nerve and serotonin in the digestive tract. It is not yet known whether taking ginger can reduce vagal activity.

Summary: Too Much or Too Little Active Vagus Nerve

In light of what has been said so far, I find it useful to make a quick summary of what happens when the Vagus Nerve is too much or too little stressed, to keep the information in order.

Not very active vagus nerve:

- Constipation, bloating, and digestive problems.
- Very high heart rate and tachycardia.
- Heaviness, stress, and anxiety.

To help:

- Meditation techniques, deep breathing, all the techniques for its activation.
- Understand what are the causes of anxiety and stress that tend to "switch off" vagal activity.
- Being able to carve out moments to unplug and dedicate to yourself.

Vagus nerve too active:

- Nausea, fainting, fatigue, very low blood pressure,
- Muscle stiffness (also present in the cervical) can affect by irritating the vagus nerve.

To help:

- Understanding the causes of muscle stiffness.

- Understand which muscle groups are involved, relieve inflammation if necessary and do specific exercises to strengthen them.

Vasovagal Syndrome: An In-Depth Study

Previously you learned briefly which situations were identified as critical by Porges, this time we deepen the topic of vasovagal syndrome a little, so as to recognize possible symptoms. This is a condition that causes the heart rate and blood pressure to drop quickly, causing the affected person to faint. This context is also referred to as vasovagal syncope or vasovagal attack; it happens more frequently in children or young adult men or women alike (Moawad and Pietrangelo, 2019). The article mentioned follows by specifying that, despite many times some causes of fainting are a sign of more important health problems, these are not usually the basis of vasovagal syndrome.

Causes

Numerous nerves are involved throughout the body to control the heartbeat and work in synergy to "administer" numerous functions such as blood pressure by controlling the width of the vessels or making sure that a sufficient quantity of oxygenated blood reaches your brain. Would you ever have said that?! In particular situations such as those leading to vasovagal syndrome, a decrease in pressure and in the amount of blood that reaches the brain is seen at the same time. Other situations that can make you pass out are:

- Get up or bend over suddenly after sitting for a long time.

- Stand for a long time.

- A heatstroke.

- Very intense physical activity.

- A sharp pain.

- Very strong and prolonged coughing fits.

Possible Symptoms

It is certainly not easy to predict fainting, but paying attention to some signs can help you understand what situation you are in.

- Have a pale or grayish appearance.

- Lightheadedness or dizziness.

- Nausea.

- Feeling sweaty or hot.

- Having a blurred vision.

- Weakness.

If these sensations are actually followed by a faint, when you recover shortly thereafter, you will feel exhausted and feel nauseous. If this has never happened to you and you suddenly experience an episode like this without apparent explanation, it is advisable to warn your doctor as there may be situations such as diabetes or cardiovascular conditions that you do not yet know at the base. Especially if you find it hard to breathe, take more than a minute to regain consciousness, are pregnant, or have problems speaking, sight or hearing. Episodes of the vasovagal syndrome do not necessarily involve the use of drugs, but it is good to understand what situations can cause them and then avoid them.

In the next section, we will learn more about foods, another fundamental component, which allows you to limit and/or avoid further inflammation in your body. This benefits both the Vagus Nerve and the functions that it performs in the viscera, and for the cervical which is often accompanied by inflammation of the muscle bands; by preferring some foods over others you will be able to have more benefits.

Food Is Your Body's Gasoline: Useful Anti-Inflammatory Foods

When it comes to food and nutrition, you really have to consider that *you become what you eat* and if a few treats occasionally are not a problem, bad habits lead to an increase in the inflammatory state of your body. The coexistence of cervical pain and a chronic inflammatory state are a typical example (Blum, 2018). In cases where the pain persists, it is worthwhile to delve into this topic and learn more about the properties of certain foods and how they can help reduce inflammation. A common process that takes place in your body is the production of free radicals, very reactive molecules or atoms that are missing an electron. When there is an excessively high amount of free radicals, these move freely in the body to try to catch the electron missing from nearby molecules. This condition is called oxidative stress and it also contributes to increasing the inflammatory state within the body. To combat it, it is useful to take foods rich in antioxidants (such as blueberries or red fruits) which give the missing electron to free radicals so as to neutralize them. The more free radicals are neutralized, the less oxidative stress and inflammation will occur. There are several possibilities to approach this issue, here are some general guidelines (you probably already know some) that you can keep in mind if you want to know, supplement or replace some foods. For specific and tailor-made information for you, always ask a professional.

- **Increase your consumption of fruit and vegetables:** Very common suggestion but do you follow it?! At least a couple of portions a day would be good, especially fruit and vegetables of

76

different colors: did you know that each color represents a different antioxidant?

- **Prefer unsaturated fats:** You can find them in olive oil, walnuts, flax seeds, almonds, sardines and bluefish, etc.; try to avoid or limit saturated fats that increase inflammation, such as cheese and butter.

- **Fish:** Fish species are rich in omega 3 (anti-inflammatory) such as salmon and sardines. Pay attention to their origin and size; in the food chain, the largest species are also those that contain the heaviest metals.

- **Limit meat:** Lean meat like chicken or turkey tends to be less inflammatory than red meat.

- **Legumes as a protein source:** hazelnuts, nuts in general, beans, and lentils are protein sources rich in antioxidants.

- **Prefer whole grains:** When you get the chance, opt for whole grain, unrefined sources. Whole grains are used to produce variations of many products such as pasta, rice, bread, and oat flakes. They are more nutritious and less inflammatory.

- **Avoid processed foods:** Preservative-rich foods are specially made to last longer but tend to have fewer nutrients and many more chemicals that contribute to inflammation. Among these, you will find sausages, carbonated drinks, baked goods, meat products, and much more.

The Effectiveness of Anti-Inflammatory Foods

At present (the article was written in 2018), there are no relevant scientific studies that show that neck pain and similar pains can be resolved without uncertainty thanks to a diet that prefers this type of food. However, there are various scientific pieces of evidence of the ability of this type of food to help reduce an inflammatory state and consequently they can be useful for reducing some types of pain such as pain resulting from obesity and arthritis; in the case of rheumatoid arthritis, benefits have been seen thanks to the Mediterranean diet.

Some Attention

Earlier it was mentioned to have precautions on the quality of the fish that is chosen taking into consideration both the origin (if farmed the quality could be lower due to the availability of limited space for their life and growth) and the size because small species will accumulate fewer toxins than larger species. Another precaution, do not to take food for good just because everyone eats it, each person may have intolerances or particular medical conditions that require different food choices.

Food for Thought: Food and Ailments

As is generally known, being careful and balancing what you eat allows you to maintain a certain level of well-being. If this topic is new to you, it may surprise you to know that your diet, some sporting activities, and maintaining a healthy weight are of great help in preventing and promoting an improvement in your well-being. The musculoskeletal system and the other elements of the back derive many benefits from certain nutritional elements that allow your body to be in shape and perform the appropriate functions. Below is an interesting list of nutrients and their benefits (Andrews, 2017):

- **Calcium:** As you may know it is a particularly important element for bone health and allows you to maintain an adequate level of bone mass throughout life and especially in old age. A correct calcium intake helps prevent the development of osteoporosis, which is painful for the vertebrae. However, calcium is not enough to strengthen bones and this is demonstrated by the high percentage of development of osteoporosis despite the high intake of this nutrient which must therefore be balanced with other nutrients for it to act in synergy. It is not only found in dairy products, but also in many legumes, leafy vegetables such as kale, salmon, and sardines, or tofu, oranges, and almonds.

  N.B. although both calcium and protein are essential for optimal bone structure, further studies will be needed to accurately determine the recommended amounts and how the two substances affect each other (Chan, 2017).

- **Magnesium:** Plays a key role in more than 300 biochemical reactions that take place in the body. If the level of magnesium in the blood drops, this is taken from the skeletal system. Its integration is useful for maintaining correct bone density and preventing back problems (if you think you can benefit from it, ask your doctor for an opinion). Magnesium is a nutrient that also helps to relax or contract the muscles, making it necessary to strengthen the muscle groups that support the spine. Magnesium can be found in green leafy vegetables, beans; fish, seeds, nuts, yogurt, dark chocolate (70% up), bananas, whole grains, and avocados.

- **Vitamin D3:** Helps the body in the absorption of calcium to create a more resistant bone structure. Without sufficient vitamin D, bones become thin, misshapen, or brittle. Vitamin D deficiency is very common and can be evidenced by blood tests. Unlike the nutrients listed so far, vitamin D is activated with the sun and is found only in certain foods such as fish (salmon is an example), cod liver oil, and egg yolks. In large retailers, you can find some products enriched with vitamin D.

- **Vitamin K2:** It is a vitamin that acts somewhat like an orchestra conductor among the minerals present in the bones. In fact, it helps distribute calcium from the soft tissues within the bone structure. It, therefore, plays an extremely important role in this metabolic function but is often very scarce and not very present in everyday diet. The synergy between K2 and calcium is therefore strategic. Vitamin K1 is the vegetable version of vitamin K, which is then converted into K2 thanks to the bacteria present in the intestine. This vitamin can be found in egg yolks, in some dairy products rather than in green leafy vegetables such as broccoli, spinach, and green cabbage.

- **Vitamin C:** It is necessary for the formation of collagen, which is the protein substance present wherever there is connective tissue, in the dermis, cartilage, ligaments, bones, and hair. It also works as an antioxidant and a correct supply of vitamin C is essential for the healing process from injured muscles, ligaments, tendons, intervertebral discs and maintains the strength of the vertebrae. You can find it easily in all fruit, as well as common vegetables like tomatoes, spinach, broccoli, or sweet potatoes.

- **Proteins:** They are an essential component of the bone structure, although they can be less considered and overshadow and favor minerals. Instead, they represent the building blocks of the body structure and serve to maintain and repair bones, cartilage, and soft tissues. Nevertheless, their importance is also central in the digestion and for various functions of the immune system.

- **Collagen:** As previously mentioned, it is a protein and constitutes up to 30% of the dry weight of the skeletal system. For this protein to form, a regular supply of amino acids and vitamin C is required.

- **Glucosamine:** It is an amino acid that can be present in high concentrations in cartilage and connective tissue. Chondroitin, on the other hand, is a substance naturally present in connective tissue and, when integrated, is often found together with glucosamine.

- **Vitamin B12:** It is a vitamin required in the formation of the bone structure and is required for the formation of healthy red blood cells in the bone marrow. The lack of this vitamin is associated with osteoporosis. You can easily find it in animal proteins such as eggs, fish, meat, and dairy products such as yogurt and cheese.

- **Iron:** It serves in the production of collagen and the conversion and activation of vitamin D. Iron is also a component of hemoglobin and myoglobin, which are two proteins responsible for transporting oxygen throughout the body, including the tissues supporting the bone marrow. An iron deficiency is not the most common but it can lead to anemia. Iron itself is not a key nutrient associated with bone "health"; however, it is an element used in other systems that are more or less directly involved in the development of the skeletal system. You can find it for example in many meat products, shellfish, red meat, poultry, green leafy vegetables, lentils, eggs, soy, whole grains, and beans.

Part 4

After learning about the anatomy of your body, you learned a little more not only about the anatomical interactions between the vertebrae of the cervical spine and the vagus nerve but also its functions, how you can activate it, and how your habits can have a more or less positive effect. I think it is useful for you to have some more resources regarding the exercises that can be done to relieve pain. Obviously, before engaging in any practice, always consult your physiotherapist or another professional figure adequately trained on the subject; however, consider the following information as a starting point to learn more about this world as well.

Things to Keep in Mind Before Performing the Exercises

Unfortunately, you may have had very acute neck pain for a couple of hours or rather a pain that increases gradually during the day. In these cases, and every time you feel pain, you would be very happy to have a magic pill that makes everything disappear. It would be certainly easier, but apart from some more or less strong painkillers, this does not exist. However, with the necessary precautions, you can have long-term benefits thanks to an exercise program that allows you, by strengthening the muscles, to support the load more easily and respond better to the stresses that your body receives every day. As Morrison (2017) specifies, relying on a trained professional guarantees you two things: having an accurate diagnosis that specifically identifies what your needs are and consequently the most suitable exercises. The second advantage is that you will be able to perform them correctly; it is not uncommon to miss some movement that leads to worsening rather than improving your condition. The cervical tract is in fact greatly influenced by other muscle groups of the upper part of the back, chest, and shoulders and some tissue massage may also be useful to complete the treatment. Often we tend to rely almost exclusively on the use of heating patches, manual massages, or similar alternatives. However, warming or relaxing the affected part is useful only for temporary relief and after a short time. These remedies can be useful and act in synergy with the exercises that you will gradually be able to do, but it is precisely the latter that in the long term allow you to be stronger and have a resistant musculature. Always remember that the exercises must never cause further pain. There may be cases where you will initially not even be able to perform the exercises, in those cases always try to reduce the inflammation first and then proceed step by step. You will see that you will gradually be able to increase flexibility as well and promote greater blood circulation to the point that is causing you problems. Strengthening the muscles allows you to protect the joints and the skeletal system from other injuries that may accidentally happen to you (McFarland, 2000).

Manual Therapy and Specific Techniques

As you may have encountered when you turn to different professionals, sometimes they look at the same problem from different points of view. A different point of view is just what I want to introduce you to today. Daul (2008), underlines a different approach common between different professionals in the sector; that is, they tend to evaluate specific exercises, for example for back problems, not necessarily as the only mode of recovery but rather as a component that acts in synergy and that is complementary to manual therapy. An example is to try to restore through manipulation the function of the sacroiliac joint (joins the iliac bone to the sacrum) affected in the case of piriformis syndrome (where the sciatic nerve is irritated by the piriformis muscle) rather than acting directly on this muscle through the specific exercise. By applying manual therapy, pressure is exerted on the muscle tissue in order to reduce tension, muscle spasms, and joint dysfunction. Overall, we can distinguish between two macro types of movement. The first focuses on the soft tissues of the muscle groups and includes massages to be able to relax the muscles, act on the scar tissue, increase circulation and decrease the pain felt. The second type, on the other hand, uses movements at different speeds and intensities (performed with more or less force) in order to release tensions in the muscles and ligaments, improve circulation and increase flexibility. When you suffer from cervical pain, very often you have more or less localized pangs also on the back that can affect more the hips or the central part. Muscle spams imply insufficiency in blood circulation and lead to three unpleasant conditions: given the poor circulation, the muscle does not receive adequate oxygenation; poor oxygenation leads the muscles to produce lactic acid and the latter makes the muscles feel sore after physical activity. Immediately after the massage, when the muscles are relaxed, lactic acid is released from the muscles and this begins to receive adequate oxygenation and blood circulation (Mueller, 2002). The next section will be entirely dedicated to this topic. Now let's briefly see some more information about some commonly used manipulative techniques (Daul, 2006):

- **Soft tissue mobilization:** It is important to understand the connection of the musculature with the ligaments. Muscle tension often decreases when correct mobilization is re-established, but sometimes this is not enough to completely eliminate spasms. In these cases, the muscle tension must be resolved at the base or the dysfunction will recur. The goal of this technique is to dissolve the fibrous tissues, move the fluid present in such a way as to relax the muscles. Once the points on which to act have been identified, these can be treated thanks to a great variety of techniques.

- **The strain counterstrain (SCS) technique:** It is an osteopathic technique that aims to correct incorrect neuromuscular reflexes that cause postural problems. Based on the point where the patient's sensitivity decreases, the therapist will be able to identify a position that will be held for 90 seconds during which a slight tension is induced. After that, you change your position allowing the body to regain its normal level of muscle tension. Since the approach is very delicate, it is indicated for those situations where the pain is very acute because the patient maintains an opposite

86

position to that in which he feels pain, thus being able to bear the treatment well.

- **Joint mobilization:** In these cases, dry ice is usually applied, and a massage or rest is recommended. While this is helpful, the relief is often only momentary and muscle spasms recur in response to joints failing to move efficiently. The person is helped to perform precisely those movements that would not be able to do alone.

- **Muscle energy techniques (METs):** They are designed ad hoc to help mobilize the joints and stretch contracted muscles. The patient must from time to time try to contract the muscles for a few seconds according to the direction set by the operator who guides him.

- **Restoration of lubrication between the joints:** This is a more direct approach than the previous two, always with the aim of helping in a correct mobilization.

So as you can see, whether you suffer from more or less severe pain, you have many means at your disposal to find relief and maintain a better long-term condition.

Cervical Spasms: What They Are and What Causes Them

You are certainly familiar with this problem and you should know that cervical spasms occur when more muscles become stiff and/or fatigued. If you have experienced a few episodes, you will know that they make activities like driving, staying focused at work, or carrying heavy objects difficult. Let's go into the specifics and learn more about this topic. They can appear suddenly or gradually; additional symptoms that may arise are (Miller, 2019):

- Throbbing pulsations.
- Fasciculation, or muscle contractions without making a real movement that occurs at regular intervals; cramps that prevent the muscles from relaxing.
- Headache before or as a consequence of the spasm.
- Blurred vision or difficulty in keeping the head erect.
- Dizziness.

The exact mechanism that leads to muscle spasm is not yet fully understood and is the subject of research; however, some elements may actually be the cause. The first case occurs when a muscle tries to protect itself from inflammation, vertebral instability, or excessive strain; or, as assumed, a muscle receives an abnormal signal from the nerve circuits or the brain (Miller, 2019). Although very often they are momentary episodes, sometimes they persist for longer and the cause to be identified can be both of psychophysical origin and connected to other pathologies. Let's see some of them (Miller, 2019):

- **Distortion, cervical trauma, tension:** In this case, the spasms are due to a protective mechanism that the muscles put in place to avoid excessive distension. A ligament injury or strain can be the cause of a muscle reflex; while the adjacent muscle fascia stiffens to protect the injured neighboring ligament.

- **Herniated disc:** In the event that proteins that contribute to increasing inflammation come out of this disc, nearby muscles can become inflamed, and in addition to causing pain, it also leads to spasms.

- **Osteoarthritis of the facet joints:** When the cartilage present begins to wear, there is friction between the vertebrae; the spurs that tend to form to stabilize the joint can help inflame and compress the nerve and cause muscle spasms.

- **Mechanical dysfunctions:** Can prevent the correct movement of the joints and give rise to spasms. These may also be due to a prolonged incorrect postural position.

- **Peripheral neuropathy:** In this case, the nerve branches that start from the spinal canal and feed the body are called peripheral nerves. If these are damaged, at the cervical level, the lesions can result in a high, low, or distorted amount of signals. This can affect many problems including motor, sensory, and even spasms.

- **Anxiety and stress:** Also in this case we find these two factors, I invite you to consider the meditation techniques proposed as a useful tool to find benefit.

- **Pain caused by myofascial syndrome:** That is inflammation and chronic pain that affects the connective tissue, therefore a muscle band located in depth. Usually, in the presence of this disorder, the cervical fascia is also affected, the musculature becomes rigid and spasms are common. The pain can increase and reach the head, and then also affect the shoulders, arms, and often the upper back when a certain point of the cervical tract is touched.

- **Cervical dystonia:** A form of torticollis marked by involuntary contractions. It can affect all age groups but is more common after the age of forty. The origin of this problem is not yet completely clear, however, a family genetic component is also assumed.

Cervical Tension: Causes and Remedies

Some more information about this aspect. It occurs in the presence of a stretch, the intensity of the pain and the extent of the affected area varies from time to time and, if the stretch usually resolves within a few days or a few weeks, the pain, on the contrary, can be prolonged over time and sometimes becoming debilitating. (Sofianos, 2017). As you have seen talking about the anatomy of the vagus nerve, of the cervical vertebrae up to these more practical aspects of the problem, you will notice the interconnection between these different facets; in fact, remember that well more than twenty muscle bands are connected to the cervical tract in a different way by the Vagus Nerve. These include the trapezius and levator scapulae muscles (I invite you to look at Figure 5). When a muscle is fully functional it is made up of numerous fibers which are in turn divided into bundles of myofibrils that contain contractile proteins, the engine of muscle contractions. When the muscles stretch too much, small tears form inside the muscle, tendon, or connective tissue and make the muscle structure weaker. The more these tears are exacerbated, the more the stretching is around the corner and, needless to say, you will need longer times to solve the problem. We just mentioned the levator scapula and trapezius muscles because it is these muscles that are most affected. The first one connects laterally the cervical spine to the scapula and plays a key role in rotating the neck laterally, a movement that is practically impossible and painful if performed in the presence of tears. Nevertheless, the trapezius reaches the shoulders and the middle of the back. The upper trapezius facilitates various movements such as tilting the head and looking upwards (Sofianos, 2017). The causes can be different and here, we find several examples of posture, or incorrect positions including holding the smartphone between the ear and shoulder while you are calling, or keeping a slightly hunched position in front of the PC. It is interesting to always bring back a shortlist of common situations, which you may know and when you see them written you consider them as obvious but in the end, it would be good to change some small habits. In fact, even lifting objects you are not used to is not beneficial; simply think of the shopping bags that you have to carry a few meters to the car when you can't find a trolley. Sofianos (2017), points out that even movements you are used to but repeated in series several times are not to be underestimated. In the lighter cases, the pain passes within a few days, while only in the most important cases it takes up to twelve weeks, therefore a good three months, to resolve definitively (Sofianos, 2017).

Daily Exercises for the Cervical Area

In this section we see some useful resources together and, in the end, I also thought of a short collection of online resources that I found particularly interesting and easy to follow. As you will have understood by reading up to here, having the constancy to carry out specific exercises helps you over time, and here are some simple instructions that can help you (Meyler, 2018):

- **Chin tuck:** It consists of making the back and head adhere to the wall and then make movements with the chin until it is lowered towards the sternum accompanied by regular breathing. Return to the initial position by raising the chin. This simple exercise helps you to strengthen the muscles that bring the head to be aligned with the shoulders.

- **Chest and levator scapula stretching:** Chest stretching exercises are very good at trying to expand the rib cage when you tend to have your shoulders hunched and projected forward. There are many exercises in this case; extend the arm horizontally along one wall and rotate the head to the opposite side to apply a slight tension between them. The levator shoulder muscle, on the other hand, is a muscle that is easily affected by trauma or injured.

If the topic is new to you, some easy-to-follow step-by-step guidelines for extending the latter may be these, proposed by (Meyler, 2018):

1. Stand up and keep your arms loose at your sides.

2. Begin by raising the right arm and bending it backward in such a way as to reach, by pushing down the right shoulder blade. (This movement allows you to rotate the scapula and help stretch the levator muscle even more before carrying out the following steps. If you have difficulty performing this step, don't worry and try the next ones.)

3. While staying in this position, try to rotate your head to the left, about 45 degrees.

4. From this position tilt your chin down so that you feel some pressure on the right side of your neck. If you had any difficulty in the second step, just try to tilt your chin sideways as reported in this fourth step.

5. If you have not experienced any difficulty, try putting your left hand behind your neck to apply more pressure and stretch the affected area further.

6. Try to stay in this position for 30–60 seconds or as long as you like.

7. Repeat on the other side.

Many people find it useful to repeat this exercise several times even when they feel that muscle stiffness is about to increase, so try to limit and "defuse" the problem. The variations of this type of exercise are numerous, however, as long as the position assumed by the shoulder does not allow it to move upwards, all the variations with which you can practice will have similar effects. Do not underestimate the benefits you can have thanks to the lengthening of this muscle band for it crosses four of the cervical vertebrae we mentioned at the beginning, specifically from the C1 vertebra (the Atlas) to the C4 vertebra, and is present on both sides of the cervical and vagus nerve. A few minutes of stretching a day can really help you lessen the tension you build up in this area. A more advanced exercise useful not only for the cervical spine but also for the upper back and shoulder blades is the cobra pose. Also known in yoga, you can perform this pose by following these steps (Morrison, 2017):

1. Grab a mat, lie on your stomach, and rest your forehead on the floor. If you prefer, you can also roll up a small towel and use it to rest your forehead.

2. Extend your arms along the floor with your palms down and place your tongue on the highest part of the palate; bring the shoulder blades towards the middle of the back and lift the hands off the floor.

3. Rotate your elbows, keep your palms up and slightly lift your forehead from the towel (if you decide to use it), and keep your gaze fixed forward.

4. Hold the position for a few seconds and then repeat several times. In this case, it is not the classic position of the cobra that keeps the palms on the ground and fully extends the arms, in this case, the upper part of the chest and the forehead are raised only partially.

In the event that these disorders were mild and did not lead you to suffer from them excessively if you are not a sportsman, consider adding a sporting activity to your routine (Gopez, 2017). Two or three hours a week is enough, don't think you have to go to the gym every day. If you are not used to it, consider the idea of starting with low-impact aerobics activities such as walking which allows you to tone the muscles in a lighter way without the need for special equipment. If you feel like it, you could use ankle or wrist weights to train your muscles more. It is an activity that you can practice both outdoors and indoors with a treadmill and it takes just half an hour of exercise for your body to start releasing endorphins, or natural analgesics. If you prefer, you can use the elliptical or the exercise bike where you can alternate steps at different speeds depending on whether you want to simulate a walk or a run; in this case, using pedals, the foot never rests on a hard surface such as asphalt, the impact of which is often reflected negatively on the well-being of the back; therefore preferring indoor activity done in this way might be the best solution. The same consideration can be done with the exercise bike by simulating cycling activity or, another valid alternative, aerobic exercises carried out in the water that combine better resistance with light impact physical activity.

Bonus: List of Online Resources

While doing research I saved some free online resources where you can follow specific exercises.

N.B. These are not sponsored links in any way, these are simply interesting resources that I want to share with you.

Some are in English: remember that if you don't know the language you can activate subtitles:

Websites

- SpineHealth.com:
  https://www.spine-health.com/conditions/neck-pain/videos

YouTube Channels

"Bob & Brad"

- Video: "10 Best Neck Pain Exercises/Stretches Ever Created"
  https://www.youtube.com/watch?v=cog4Dds_a0

- Video: "Tight & Painful Neck? 2 NEVER Do Exercises & 3 BEST Exercises"
  https://www.youtube.com/watch?v=1UF_HYBCh_Q

- Video: "Most Important Exercises to Help Pinched Nerve & Neck Pain"
  https://www.youtube.com/watch?v=RdgDg9_SL48

- Video: "How to Get Rid of Muscle Knots in Traps, Shoulder and Back in 90 seconds"
  https://www.youtube.com/watch?v=23ZWC5EgdLs

- Video "Eight Everyday Habits Harming Your Spine (Neck & Back)"
  https://www.youtube.com/watch?v=KFTI2PHgRIA

"The Yoga Monkey"

- Video: Yoga – "Exercises for the neck and shoulders"
  https://www.youtube.com/watch?v=cDHQGVU5Tsw

"The Other Rehabilitation"

- Playlist video: "Cervical disorder: insights and exercises"
  https://www.youtube.com/playlist?list=PLe2hVDv1kjq-c-an6GubyZZ7A_i7n4yob

Conclusion

Here we are at the end of this journey! I hope you enjoyed it and you now have the tools to better understand what is happening to you. We started by understanding why the cervical is different from other forms of pain and the intricate connections that are present between the skull, the upper back, when and how the different muscle bands come into play, and how seven vertebrae can support your head. Many different functions, but as in nature, your body is also an ecosystem that is characterized by the complexity and synergy of different functions. You have understood the functions of the Vagus Nerve, how to activate it and how it allows you to relax and make it easier for you to release the tension that you accumulate every day at work or in the family. In the management of emotions different branches of the nervous system come into play, some more archaic, others more modern but all of them, if activated at the right time, allow you to live better. Don't neglect the nutritional part: food is your body's gasoline, and its quality makes the difference and reduces the inflammations that are easily created. In addition to the practice of meditation and relaxation, excellent for both the cervical and the activation of the Vagus Nerve, it is important to strengthen the cervical muscles to strengthen the muscles that will become excellent tools in everyday activities, so take a look also to the video bonuses that I shared on the last page.

Thank you for coming this far and I hope you appreciated the notions that I have collected and organized for you. I wanted to provide you with scientific-based information in order to help you better orient yourself among the tide of information you find online.

See you soon!

—*Emma.*

Bibliography

A.Rosenkranz, M., J.Davidson, R., G.MacCoo, D., F.Sheridan, J., H.Kalin, N., & Lutz, A. (Volume 27, January 2013, Pages 174–184.). *A Comparison of Mindfulness-Based Stress Reduction and an Active control in Modulation of Neurogenic Inflammation*. Tratto da Brain, Behavior, and Immunity: https://www.sciencedirect.com/science/article/abs/pii/S088915 9112004758

Andrews, K. (2017). *Food for Thought: Diet and Nutrition for a Healthy Back*. Tratto da SPINE-health: https://www.spine-health.com/wellness/nutrition-diet-weight-loss/food-thought-diet-and-nutrition-a-healthy-back

Author, U. (2021). *The Journal of Psychological Sciences*. Taken from State of Mind magazine: https://www.stateofmind.it/tag/teoria-polivagale/

Author, U. (s.d.). *Relaxation Techniques*. Taken from Cognitive Studies: https://studicognitivi.it/tecnica/tecniche-di-rilassamento/ Consulted in May 2021.

Bernardi L, S. P.-S. (2001, PMID: 11751348; PMCID: PMC61046.). Effect of Rosary Prayer and Yoga Mantras on Autonomic Cardiovascular Rhythms: A Comparative Study. . *BMJ. 2001 Dec 22–*

29;323(7327):1446–9. DOI: 10.1136/bmj.323.7327.1446., p. https://pubmed.ncbi.nlm.nih.gov/11751348/.

Block, A. (2007). *11 Chronic Pain Control Techniques.* Tratto da SPINE-health: https://www.spine-health.com/conditions/chronic-pain/11-chronic-pain-control-techniques

Blum, S. M. (2018). *Anti-Inflammatory Foods to Try for Neck Pain.* Tratto da SPINE-health: https://www.spine-health.com/conditions/neck-pain/anti-inflammatory-foods-try-neck-pain

Bravo JA, F. P. (2011; Epub 2011 Aug 29. PMID: 21876150; PMCID: PMC3179073.). *Ingestion of Lactobacillus Strain Regulates Emotional Behavior and Central GABA Receptor Expression in a Mouse Via the Vagus Nerve. . Proc Natl Acad Sci U S A. 2011 Sep 20;108(38):16050–5. doi:10.1073/pnas.1102999108.* , p. https://pubmed.ncbi.nlm.nih.gov/21876150/.

Breit, S., Kupferberg, A., Rogler, G., & Hasler, G. (2018). *Vagus Nerve as Modulator of the Brain-Gut Axis in Psychiatric and Inflammatory Disorders. Front Psychiatry. 9:44.*, https://www.ncbi.nlm.nih.gov/pmc/articles/PMC5859128/.

C., V. S. (2(3):251–62. doi: 10.2147/vhrm.2006.2.3.251. PMID: 17326331; PMCID: PMC1993981.). *A Review of Omega-3 Ethyl Esters for Cardiovascular Prevention and Treatment of Increased Blood Triglyceride Levels. Vasc Health Risk Manag. 2006;*, p. https://pubmed.ncbi.nlm.nih.gov/17326331/.

Cearley, S. M., Immaneni, S., & Shankar., P. (2017. Pages 117–121). *Irritable Bowel Syndrome: The Effect of FODMAPs and Meditation on Pain Management. European Journal of Integrative Medicine. Volume 12.*, p. https://www.sciencedirect.com/science/article/abs/pii/S187638 2017301014.

Chan, T. (s.d.). *Calcium: What's Best for Your Bones and health?* From Harvard School of Public Health. : http://www.hsph.harvard.edu. Accessed March 1, 2017.

Chiapponi, M. (s.d.). From Laltrariabilitazione: https://www.laltrariabilitazione.it/category/cervicale-articoli.

Chiapponi, M. (2021, Maggio). *Vagus Nerve: The Key to Improving Many Symptoms and Ailments?* From https://www.laltrariabilitazione.it/cervicale-articoli/nervo-vago-la-chiave-migliorare-molti-sintomi-disturbi.html

Cohen, J., Ritter, J., & Aleksic, A. (2021). *19 Factors That May Stimulate Your Vagus Nerve Naturally. SelfHacked*, p. https://selfhacked.com/blog/32-ways-to-stimulate-your-vagus-nerve-and-all-you-need-to-know-about-it/.

Daul, R. (2006). *Specific Manual Physical Therapy Techniques. SPINE-health*, p. https://www.spine-health.com/treatment/physical-therapy/specific-manual-physical-therapy-techniques.

Deardorff, W. (2017). *Understanding Chronic Pain.* Tratto da SPINE-health: https://www.spine-health.com/conditions/chronic-pain/understanding-chronic-pain

Dickerman, R. (2019). *C1-C2 Treatment.* Tratto da SPINE-health: https://www.spine-health.com/conditions/spine-anatomy/c1-c2-treatment

Dickerman, R. D. (2019). *The C1-C2 Vertebrae and Spinal Segment.* Tratto da SPINE-health: https://www.spine-health.com/conditions/spine-anatomy/c1-c2-vertebrae-and-spinal-segment

Encyclopedia., B. B. (2018). *Headache. Encyclopedia Britannica.* https://www.britannica.com/science/headache. Consulted: May 2021.

Gopez, J. (2017). *Low-Impact Aerobic Exercise. SPINE-health,* p. https://www.spine-health.com/wellness/exercise/low-impact-aerobic-exercise.

Goyal M, S. S.-S. (2014). *Meditation Programs for Psychological Stress and Well-Being: A Systematic Review and Meta-Analysis.* Tratto da JAMA Intern Med. : https://pubmed.ncbi.nlm.nih.gov/24395196/

Gross, K. (2018). *Cervical Vertigo.* Tratto da Healthline: https://www.healthline.com/health/cervical-vertigo

Howland, R. (2015). *Vagus Nerve Stimulation.* Tratto da PMC. US National Library of Medicine. National Institutes of Health.: https://www.ncbi.nlm.nih.gov/pmc/articles/PMC4017164/

Ingraham, P. (2021, May). *Does Posture Matter? A Detailed Guide to Posture and Postural Correction Strategies (Especially Why None of It Matters Very*

Much). Tratto da https://www.painscience.com/articles/posture.php

Innis, J. M. (Accessed: June 2021). *Calming a Wigged Out Autonomic Nervous System Using the Vagus Nerve. Innis Integrative Bodymind Therapy*, p. https://www.innisintegrativetherapy.com/blog/2017/11/21/cal ming-a-wigged-out-autonomic-nervous-system-using-the-vagus-nerve.

Jacobson, E. (s.d.). *Progressive Relaxation. University of Chicago Press.* Tratto da Consultato nel sito web: Studi Cognitivi: https://studicognitivi.it/tecnica/tecniche-di-rilassamento/

Jason C. Ong, P. R. (1 September 2014, Pages 1553–1563., https://doi.org/10.5665/sleep.4010). *A Randomized Controlled Trial of Mindfulness Meditation for Chronic Insomnia. Sleep, Volume 37, Issue 9.*

Kiken, L. G. (2014). Does Mindfulness Attenuate Thoughts Emphasizing Negativity, but Not Positivity? *Journal of Research in Personality Vol. 53 (2014): 22–30*, p. doi:10.1016/j.jrp.2014.08.002.

Kok BE, C. K. (Epub 2013 May 6. Erratum in: Psychol Sci. 2016 Jun;27(6):931. PMID: 23649562.). *How Positive Emotions Build Physical Health: Perceived Positive Social Connections Account for the Upward Spiral Between Positive Emotions and Vagal Tone. Psychol Sci. 2013 Jul 1;24(7):1123–32. doi: 10.1177/0956797612470827.*, p. https://pubmed.ncbi.nlm.nih.gov/23649562/.

Laine Green A, W. D. (doi: 10.1016/j.jocn.2013.03.017. Epub 2013 Aug 17. PMID: 23962632.). *Vagal Stimulation by Manual Carotid Sinus*

Massage to Acutely Suppress Seizures. . J Clin Neurosci. 2014 Jan;21(1):179–80., p. https://pubmed.ncbi.nlm.nih.gov/23962632/.

Lanska, D. J. (2002; 58:452–459). *Corning and Vagal Nerve Stimulation for Seizures in the 1880s. Neurology.* https://pubmed.ncbi.nlm.nih.gov/11839848/.

Lara Hilton, A. R. (2017). *Meditation for Posttraumatic Stress: Systematic Review and Meta-Analysis. Psychol Trauma. 2017 Jul; 9(4):453–460.* , p. doi: 10.1037/tra0000180. Epub 2016 Aug 18. PMID: 27537781.

Leanage, N. (2020, Agosto). *The Vagus Nerve (CN X).* Tratto da MedScape: https://emedicine.medscape.com/article/1875813-overview#a1

Levine, J. (2019). *All About the C6-C7 Spinal Motion Segment.* Tratto da SPINE-health: https://www.spine-health.com/conditions/spine-anatomy/all-about-c6-c7-spinal-motion-segment

Mansoor M. Aman, R. J. (2018 Apr 4;22(5):33.). *Evidence-Based Non-Pharmacological Therapies for Fibromyalgia. Curr Pain Headache Rep.*, p. doi: 10.1007/s11916–018–0688–2. PMID: 29619620.

Mason H, V. M. (Epub 2013 Apr 23. PMID: 23710236; PMCID: PMC3655580.). *Cardiovascular and Respiratory Effect of Yogic Slow Breathing in the Yoga Beginner: What Is the Best Approach?* Evid Based Complement Alternat. *Med. 2013;2013:743504. doi: 10.1155/2013/743504.* , p. https://pubmed.ncbi.nlm.nih.gov/23710236/.

McFarland Ph.D. PT, C. (2000). *How a Physical Therapist Can Help with Exercise.* *SPINE-health,* p. https://www.spine-health.com/treatment/spine-specialists/how-a-physical-therapist-can-help-exercise.

Meyler, Z. (2018). *Easy Levator Scapulae Stretch for Neck Pain. SPINE-health,* p. https://www.spine-health.com/wellness/exercise/easy-levator-scapulae-stretch-neck-pain.

Meyler, Z. (2019). *C2-C5 Treatment.* From SPINE-health: https://www.spine-health.com/conditions/spine-anatomy/c2-c5-treatment

Meyler, Z. D. (2018). *Daily Exercises and Stretches to Prevent Neck Pain. SPINE-health,* p. https://www.spine-health.com/wellness/exercise/daily-exercises-and-stretches-prevent-neck-pain.

Meyler, Z. D. (2019). *All About the C2-C5 Spinal Motion Segments.* From SPINE-health: https://www.spine-health.com/conditions/spine-anatomy/all-about-c2-c5-spinal-motion-segments

Miller, M. a. (2009). *"The Effect of Mirthful Laughter on the Human Cardiovascular System.". Medical Hypotheses Vol. 73,5 (2009): 636–9. doi:10.1016/j.mehy.2009.02.044,* p. https://www.ncbi.nlm.nih.gov/pmc/articles/PMC2814549/.

Miller, R. (2019). *Understanding Neck Spasms. SPINE-health,* p. https://www.spine-health.com/conditions/neck-pain/understanding-neck-spasms.

Miller, R. P. (2019). *What Causes Neck Spasms? SPINE-health*, p. https://www.spine-health.com/conditions/neck-pain/what-causes-neck-spasms.

Morrison Gavin, P. (2017). *What to Consider Before Starting Exercises for Neck Pain. SPINE-health.*

Morrison, G. (2017). *Neck Strengthening Exercises. SPINE-health*, p. https://www.spine-health.com/conditions/neck-pain/neck-strengthening-exercises.

Morrison, G. P. (2018). *Forward Head Posture's Effect on Neck Muscles.* From SPINE-health: https://www.spine-health.com/conditions/neck-pain/forward-head-postures-effect-neck-muscles. Consulted: May 2021

MPT, D. R. (2006). *Manual Physical Therapy for Pain Relief. SPINE-health*, p. https://www.spine-health.com/treatment/physical-therapy/manual-physical-therapy-pain-relief.

Mueller, B. R. (2002). *Neuromuscular Massage Therapy. SPINE-health*, p. https://www.spine-health.com/wellness/massage-therapy/neuromuscular-massage-therapy.

Nguyen, K. (2019). *What Causes Neck Pain and Dizziness?* From SPINE-health: https://www.spine-health.com/conditions/neck-pain/what-causes-neck-pain-and-dizziness

Nicole, S. (consulted may 2021). *Radicolopatia Cervicale: Diagnosi e Trattamento.* Tratto da Fisio Science:

https://www.fisioscience.it/blog/radicolopatia-cervicale-diagnosi-e-trattamento/

Olex S, N. A. (Epub 2013 Jul 24. PMID: 23890919.). *Meditation: Should a Cardiologist Care? Int J Cardiol. 2013 Oct 3;168(3):1805–10. doi: 10.1016/j.ijcard.2013.06.086.*

Pietrangelo Ann. (2019; Medically reviewed by Heidi Moawad, M.D.). *Everything You Need to Know About Vasovagal Syncope. healthline*, p. https://www.healthline.com/health/vasovagal-syncope.

Reiley , A., Vickory, F., Funderburg, S., Cesario, R., & Clendaniel, R. (2017). *Cervicogenic Dizziness.* From VEDA: https://vestibular.org/article/diagnosis-treatment/types-of-vestibular-disorders/cervicogenic-dizziness/

Ruffoli, R., Giorgi, F., & Pizzanelli, C. (2011;42:288–296.). *The Chemical Neuroanatomy of Vagus Nerve Stimulation. . J Chem Neuroanatomy.* https://pubmed.ncbi.nlm.nih.gov/21167932/.

Sofianos, D. (2017). *Neck Strain: Causes and Remedies. SPINE-health*, p. https://www.spine-health.com/conditions/neck-pain/neck-strain-causes-and-remedies.

Sood A, J. D. (2013). *On Mind Wandering, Attention, Brain Networks, and Meditation. Explore (NY). 2013 May-Jun;9(3):136–41. doi:10.1016/j.explore.2013.02.005. PMID: 23643368.*

Thorpe, M., & Link, R. (Medically reviewed by Marney A. White, Ph.D., MS. Updated on October 27, 2020). *12 Science-Based Benefits of*

Meditation.   From   Healthline.   :
https://www.healthline.com/nutrition/12-benefits-of-meditation

Traynelis, V. C. (2020). *Upper Cervical Spine Disorders: Anatomy of the Head and Upper Neck. A Quick Lesson to Help You Learn More About Your Craniovertebral Junction Condition.* From Spine Universe: https://www.spineuniverse.com/conditions/upper-neck-disorders/upper-cervical-spine-disorders-anatomy-head-upper-neck

Vickhoff B, M. H. (Published 2013 Jul 9. doi:10.3389/fpsyg.2013.00334, [published correction appears in Front Psychol. 2013 Sep 05;4:599].). *Music Structure Determines Heart Rate Variability of Singers. Front Psychol. 2013;4:334.*   ,   p. https://www.ncbi.nlm.nih.gov/pmc/articles/PMC3705176/.

Zigler, J. M. (2018). *All About the C5-C6 Spinal Motion Segment.* From SPINE-health: https://www.spine-health.com/conditions/spine-anatomy/all-about-c5-c6-spinal-motion-segment